AN INTRODUCTION TO ISSUES IN COMMUNITY HEALTH NURSING IN CANADA

AN INTRODUCTION TO ISSUES IN COMMUNITY HEALTH NURSING IN CANADA

Janet Ross Kerr, RN, PhD
Professor
Faculty of Nursing
University of Alberta
Edmonton, Alberta

Jannetta MacPhail, MSN, PhD, LLD (Hon)
Professor Emeritus
Faculty of Nursing
University of Alberta
Edmonton, Alberta

Mosby

St. Louis Baltimore Boston
Carlsbad Chicago Naples New York Philadelphia Portland
London Madrid Mexico City Singapore Sydney Tokyo Toronto Wiesbaden

Mosby
Dedicated to Publishing Excellence

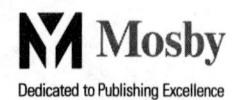

A Times Mirror Company

Publisher: Nancy L. Coon
Editor: Loren Wilson
Developmental Editor: Brian Dennison
Project Manager: Carol Sullivan Weis
Designer: Sheilah Barrett

A NOTE TO THE READER:
The author and publisher have made every attempt to check dosages and nursing content for accuracy. Because the science of pharmacology is continually advancing, our knowledge base continues to expand. Therefore we recommend that the reader always check product information for changes in dosage or administration before administering any medication. This is particularly important with new or rarely used drugs.

Copyright © 1996 by Mosby–Year Book, Inc.

All rights reserved. No part of this publication may be reproduced, stored in a retrieval system, or transmitted, in any form or by any means, electronic, mechanical, photocopying, recording, or otherwise, without prior written permission from the publisher.

Permission to photocopy or reproduce solely for internal or personal use is permitted for libraries or other users registered with the Copyright Clearance Center, provided that the base fee of $4.00 per chapter plus $.10 per page is paid directly to the Copyright Clearance Center, 27 Congress Street, Salem, MA 01970. This consent does not extend to other kinds of copying, such as copying for general distribution, for advertising or promotional purposes, for creating new collected works, or for resale.

Printed in the United States of America
Composition by Top Graphics
Printing and binding by Plus Communications

Mosby–Year Book, Inc.
11830 Westline Industrial Drive
St. Louis, Missouri 63146

International Standard Book Number 0-8151-4930-1

96 97 98 99 00 / 9 8 7 6 5 4 3 2 1

PREFACE

The horizons of community health are rapidly changing as a new hard line on health spending by provincial and federal governments has centred on downsizing the large and powerful acute care segment of the Canadian health care system. One outcome of this downsizing has been renewed interest in the community sector with a concomitant shift in focus to give health care consumers more authority and responsibility for managing their own health care. Although the political agenda has fuelled the reform movement, it remains to be seen whether long-term outcomes are driven by political ideology or a more grass roots approach to the promotion and maintenance of health. Nurses are at the centre of the reform movement. Ironically, at the same time, nurses are being displaced in large numbers from the acute-care system, they are being seen as key front-line professionals in a community-based health strategy. As the system gears up to develop a much stronger community orientation to health, nurses have found themselves in pivotal and important roles providing health care, which could not otherwise be delivered to those who require it. The future is bright for community health nursing in Canada and as the parameters of the health system change to accommodate new ideas about how health care should be delivered, it is likely that nurses will play major roles at the practice, administrative, and policy levels.

An Introduction to Issues in Community Health Nursing in Canada addresses a broad range of issues in community health arising within the Canadian health system. In defining the scope of the book, we have attempted to concentrate on issues that characterize nursing in the community from a Canadian perspective. The historical stage on which community health nursing in Canada developed has been outlined in the first chapter. An analysis of the Canadian health care system follows in terms of the fundamental assumptions on which it is based and the way in which it has evolved over time. Two chapters on primary health care of communities and primary health care of families provide a perspective on community health care at various levels in the community. An understanding of ethical and legal issues in health care is essential for all practitioners; an overview of important ethical and legal issues in nursing practice is presented in Chapter 5. The book concludes with an analysis of major challenges facing the profession in general and community health nursing in particular in Canada in relation to practice, education, and research.

We hope that the content of this book will be helpful to students studying community health nursing in undergraduate nursing programs in Canada. Through teaching trends and issues in nursing in Canada to undergraduate and graduate nursing students at the University of Alberta, we have found that the development of a primary health care approach to community health gives rise to very exciting possibilities. Primary health care has the potential to redefine the health system, and many changes are currently taking place in the organization of health care in Canada. A major goal of primary health care is the empowerment of individuals, families, and communities. This empowerment is potentially the most important development in health care within the past 4 decades. We are most interested in responses of readers to this book and welcome feedback from any interested readers. We can be reached through correspondence addressed to us at the University of Alberta (3rd floor, Faculty of Nursing, University of Alberta, Edmonton, Alberta, Canada T6 G 1T6).

Janet Ross Kerr
Jannetta MacPhail

Acknowledgments

We would like to express our appreciation to the following authors who contributed a chapter to this book:

Margaret Harrison, RN, PhD
Professor
Faculty of Nursing
The University of Alberta
Edmonton, Alberta

Linda Reutter, RN, PhD
Associate Professor
Faculty of Nursing
The University of Alberta
Edmonton, Alberta

We would also like to thank the following reviewers who read the manuscript for this book:

Diane Gamble
Okanagan University College
Kelowna, British Columbia

Lynnette Leeseberg Stamler
University of Windsor
Windsor, Ontario

Peggy Morrison
Canadore College
North Bay, Ontario

CONTENTS

1   THE GROWTH OF COMMUNITY HEALTH NURSING IN CANADA, 1
    Janet Ross Kerr

2   THE SHAPE AND STRUCTURE OF HEALTH CARE IN CANADA, 16
    Janet Ross Kerr

3   PRIMARY HEALTH CARE AND THE HEALTH OF COMMUNITIES, 29
    Jannetta MacPhail

4   PRIMARY HEALTH CARE AND THE HEALTH OF FAMILIES, 46
    Linda Reutter and Margaret Harrison

5   ETHICAL AND LEGAL QUESTIONS IN NURSING PRACTICE, 59
    Jannetta MacPhail and Janet Ross Kerr

6   NURSING RESEARCH AS A BASIS FOR PRACTICE IN COMMUNITY HEALTH NURSING, 81
    Jannetta MacPhail

7   CURRENT AND FUTURE CHALLENGES IN COMMUNITY HEALTH NURSING, 97
    Janet Ross Kerr and Jannetta MacPhail

An Introduction to Issues in Community Health Nursing in Canada

1

THE GROWTH OF COMMUNITY HEALTH NURSING IN CANADA

JANET ROSS KERR

The roots of public health and public health nursing in Canada can be traced to the settlements of New France in the seventeenth and eighteenth centuries. The concept of caring for the sick and the poor was central to Christian beliefs about the relationship between the body and the spirit, and these ideas were reflected in the missionary zeal of Roman Catholic religious orders in New France. Women had been primary caregivers to the sick and needy in the community in France, and French religious congregations that attracted women of social standing to membership offered nursing services in hospitals and the community. Indeed, caring in the community for the sick and the poor had legitimately fallen within the scope of women's roles in society for centuries, and as hostels, hospitals, and orphanages were developed, caregiving for those who required these services also became the domain of women. The traditions within which nursing developed in Canada formed the basis for the care given to native people, fur traders, and eventually settlers.

The importance of class differentials in the development of modern public health services in Canada had been pointed out by Boutilier. Philanthropy and helping were closely associated with the upper and middle class strata of society, while the recipients of that assistance were clearly members of the lower socioeconomic groups who needed the basic essentials of life. Women have been important in achieving societal goals involving philanthropic and altruistic objectives, and this has been reflected strongly in nursing organizations over time. As nursing developed as a profession for lay women in Canada from the 1870s on, mothering and domesticity remained the link from the home and the women's movement into the world of professional nursing. Women's associations became the key players in the public health crusade in Canada. As the National Council of Women embraced a professional standard of education for nurses in Canada in 1898 and approved the formation of the Victorian Order of Nurses, they did so not only on the basis of the need to acquire essential knowledge for nursing but also on the basis of the fundamental attributes that nurses as women were believed to share with all women, that is, altruism, philanthropy, and moral duty (Boutilier, pp. 41-42).

■ Early Nursing in New France

Similar values are associated with early nursing in New France. It should be recognized that in tracing the roots of the European settlements in the new world, there is a tendency to forget that there were thousands of native people living on the North American continent before the European migration. The native peoples had their own informal health system, as well as natural herbal remedies for various ailments. The first European nurses to tend the sick were male attendants at a "sick bay" established at the French garrison in Port Royal in Acadia in 1629 (Gibbon and Mathewson, 1947). The Jesuit priests, who were the first missionaries to emigrate to New France, encountered the need to care for the sick in pursuing their primary goal to convert the natives to Christianity. The Jesuits travelled to the native villages where they ministered to the sick as they put forth their religious teachings. Because the body and the soul were seen as inseparable, their efforts to relieve bodily distress assisted them in their religious work (Parkman, 1897, p. 176).

The first lay woman who regularly cared for the sick, both in her home and in other homes in the community, was Marie Rollet, married to the surgeon-apothecary, Louis Hébert. The Hébert family emigrated to Quebec in 1617 at the request of Champlain. Louis Hébert had previous experience in the New World, having made journeys to Île St. Croix in 1604 to 1605 and to Port Royal in 1606 to 1607 and 1610 to 1613. On his fourth journey, he embarked from Honfleur in 1617 accompanied by Mme Hébert and their three children. Mme Marie Hébert thus became the first woman to emigrate from France to the new colony in what was to become Canada (Brown, 1966). In Quebec, Louis Hébert's "apothecary skill and his small store of grain were a godsend to the sick and starving winterers. In spite of the company's demands on his and his servant's time, he succeeded in clearing and planting some land" (Brown, 1966, p. 368). "Marie Rollet aided her husband in caring for the sick and shared his interest in the savages" (Brown, 1966, p. 578). This was quite natural, since it was common practice for French wives of the early seventeenth century to collaborate with their husbands in their work. Of special attention was Mme Hébert's genuine concern for the indigenous people as intelligent human beings. The efforts of Mme Hébert and her husband to care for the natives and share health knowledge with them appear to have been welcomed and appreciated (Thwaites, 1959).

The *Jesuit Relations* were informative reports written regularly by the Jesuit missionary priests for public relations purposes because they needed support on a regular basis. This information was widely circulated and the French people learned about New France in this way. The *Relations* were written over a 72-year period and provide a marvellous account of life in early Canada. "It was clear to the fathers that their ministrations were valued solely because their religion was supposed by many to be a 'medicine' or charm, efficacious against disease and death" (Parkman, 1897, p. 179). Thus they sent urgent requests for nurses to come to the colony to assist with their work. In 1634 Father LeJeune wrote in his *Relation:*

> If we had a hospital here, all the sick people of the country, and all the old people, would be there. As to the men, we will take care of them according to our means; but, in regard to the women, it is not becoming for us to receive them into our houses (Kenton, 1925, p. 49).

Propriety did not allow the Jesuit priests to treat native women who were ill on their premises. This presented another pressing reason for female members of a nursing order to come to Canada to assist with the work. It is somewhat curious to reflect on the fact that "Quebec, as we have seen, had a seminary, a hospital, and a convent, before it had a population" (Parkman, 1897, p. 259).

■ Hospitalières de la Miséricorde de Jésus

The Duchesse d'Aiguillon, a niece of Cardinal Richelieu, read and was moved by the *Relations* and developed a plan to build the Hôtel Dieu at Québec. She used her influence to obtain a grant of land and arranged for the careful selection of three nuns of the Hospitalières de la Miséricorde de Jésus to go to Canada to establish the hospital. The three nuns, who all came from good families, were Marie Guenet de St. Ignace (later Mére de St. Ignace), Anne Lecointre de St. Bernard, and Marie Forestier de St. Bonaventure de Jésus. Aboard ship at Dieppe the "hospital nuns" encountered three Ursuline nuns, whose mission was to teach the natives, and Madame de la Peltrie, who intended to help establish a convent school for the native children. The voyage was perilous, lasting from May to August 1639 (Juchereau and Duplessis, 1939). Upon their arrival the women began work immediately:

> The Hospital Nuns arrived at Kebec on the first day of August of last year. Scarcely had they disembarked before they found themselves overwhelmed with patients. The hall of the hospital being too small, it was necessary to erect some cabins, fashioned like those of the savages, in their garden. Not having furniture for so many people, they had to cut in two or three pieces part of the blankets and sheets they had brought for these poor sick people (Kenton, 1925, p. 157).

As there was no time to make any preparations, the nuns had to throw themselves into their work from the first day:

> ... instead of taking a little rest and refreshing themselves after the great discomforts they had suffered upon the sea, they found themselves so burdened and occupied that we had fear of losing them and their hospital at its very birth. The sick came from all directions in such numbers, their stench was so insupportable, the heat so great, the fresh food so

scarce and so poor, in a country so new and strange, that I do not know how these good sisters, who almost had not even leisure in which to take a little sleep, endured all these hardships (Kenton, 1925, p. 157).

The smallpox epidemic, which was raging on the sisters' arrival and for a considerable length of time thereafter, also required the labours of the Ursuline nuns, whose school convent became a hospital "and they found themselves nursing instead of teaching" (Millman, 1965, p. 424). Jamieson commented on the fact that the Ursulines used native Indian women for assistance in their hospitals and that "their teacher training was instrumental in providing the earliest instruction and supervision of nurses in America" (Jamieson, Sewall, and Gjertson, 1959, p. 196).

New recruits from Dieppe were sought, and the first two arrived the following summer. But by 1671 the nuns were obtaining sufficient local recruits to the order and no longer depended on assistance from France. The archives of the Hôtel Dieu of Quebec contain a letter from Vincent de Paul written in April, 1652: "I consider this enterprise as one of the greatest accomplishments within fifteen hundred years" (Gibbon and Mathewson, 1947, p. 15). Several additions were constructed to their facility as the need arose. One epidemic after another often brought more patients to their doorstep than they could accommodate. The worst appears to have been a smallpox epidemic in 1703, when more than a quarter of the nuns died:

> Our sisters fell ill in such numbers from the very first that there were not enough of those who were well to look after the infected cases in our rooms and wards. We accepted the offer of service from several good widows (Gibbon and Mathewson, 1947, p. 35).

Jeanne Mance

La Société de Notre Dame de Jésus was composed of a group of philanthropists who wanted to establish a colony of a religious character to work with the Indians on the Island of Montreal. This was no easy matter because they had to secure the charter for the land and raise sufficient funds to send a carefully selected group of people to create the society they had in mind. Jeanne Mance had read the *Jesuit Relations* regularly and believed she had been called to serve in the New World. Through the wealth of Mme de Bullion, Jeanne Mance was asked to take charge of building a hospital in the settlement that was to be established at Montreal. Thus she sailed from La Rochelle, along with 3 women and 40 men, under the leadership of Paul de Chomédy, Sieur de Maisonneuve (Canadian Nurses Association [CNA], 1968). Their two ships arrived in Quebec, but their reception was not a welcoming one. They:

> ... arrived too late in the season to ascend to Montreal before winter. They encountered distrust, jealousy, and opposition. The agents of the Company of the Hundred Associates looked on them askance; and the Governor of Quebec, Montmagny, saw a rival governor

in Maisonneuve. Every means was used to persuade the adventurers to abandon their project, and settle at Quebec (Parkman, 1897, p. 296).

Steadfast in his resolve to accomplish the mission to establish a settlement at Montreal, Maisonneuve "expressed his surprise that they should assume to direct his affairs. 'I have not come here,' he said, 'to deliberate, but to act. It is my duty and my honour to found a colony at Montreal; and I would go, if every tree were an Iroquois!'" (Parkman, 1897, pp. 296-297). The group had difficulty finding housing for the winter, but through the generosity of one colonist, they were housed at St. Michel. Jeanne Mance found that her neighbors were the hospital nuns who lived in their mission at Sillery, not far from Quebec. Here Jeanne Mance spent a good deal of her time assisting in the work of the hospital, and this undoubtedly served her well as she ventured to Montreal as the only person with health-care knowledge.

On May 17, 1642 when Maisonneuve and his followers landed at Montreal, the Associates of Montreal took possession of the land that "Champlain, thirty-one years before, had chosen as the fit site of a settlement" (Parkman, 1897, p. 302). They gave thanks, then proceeded to establish their settlement. The hospital was one of the first buildings constructed in the colony, although there were apparently some misgivings:

> It is true that the hospital was not wanted as no one was sick at Ville Marie and one or two chambers would have sufficed for every prospective necessity; but it will be remembered that the colony had been established in order that a hospital might be built . . . Instead then of tilling the land to supply their own pressing needs, all labourers of the settlement were set at this pious though superfluous task (Parkman, 1897, p. 362).

All of the new settlers were committed to the objective of converting the Indians to Christianity and sought to gain their favour in whatever way they could. "If they could persuade them to be nursed, they were consigned to the tender care of Mlle Mance" (Parkman, 1897, p. 364).

As she was soon in need of more help than the one young girl who had come with her, Jeanne Mance enlisted the assistance of two others to cope with the patient load. She made three trips back to France, one 4 years after her arrival, one in 1657, and one in 1663. All of these trips were made primarily for the purpose of meeting with members of the Associates of Notre Dame of Montreal and other benefactors to generate resources for her hospital. She also arranged for assistance in her hospital from a nursing order in France in 1659. Thus three nuns of St. Joseph de la Flèche arrived to assist in nursing the sick in her hospital, of which she remained the administrator. When she died in 1673, she was "universally respected and beloved by the Colony which she had helped to found" (Gibbon and Mathewson, 1947, p. 30). The highest award of the Canadian Nurses Association, the Jeanne Mance Award, is named in honour of this famous Canadian nurse.

The Grey Nuns of Montreal

The Grey Nuns of Montreal are considered the first visiting nurses in Canada. This uniquely Canadian order of nuns was formed in 1738 by Marguerite d'Youville, a widow who was a niece of the explorer, La Vérendrye. This was also the first non-cloistered order to be established in Canada, patterned after the model initiated by St. Vincent de Paul. Mme d'Youville organized this group of women with charitable intentions, and they "agreed to combine their possessions in a house of refuge chiefly for the poor, taking the names of Soeurs Grises or Grey Nuns" (Gibbon and Mathewson, 1947, p. 45).

Because they had to raise funds to subsist and carry on their work with the sick and the poor, the Grey Nuns had to struggle to make ends meet. For the purpose of raising money, wealthy paying guests were taken in, and the sisters did handiwork that they sold. Because the order was not cloistered and because it took up the nursing of patients in their homes, something not previously done in New France, there was originally some mistrust of its work and intentions. "Though they usually did their visiting in pairs for self-protection, the Grey Nuns were innovators and subject to misunderstanding" (Gibbon and Mathewson, 1947, p. 46). It is important to recognize that the other orders of nuns, the Augustinians in Quebec and the St. Joseph's Hospitallers of Montreal, were cloistered and were not permitted to venture into the community except in an emergency by special permission of the Bishop.

A fire in 1745 destroyed their house, and the Grey Nuns were forced to move from one place to another for the next 2 years to carry on their work. Then the Gentlemen of Saint Sulpice gave permission for Madame d'Youville and the Grey Nuns to take over the General Hospital under a charter as the Soeurs de la Charité de l'Hôspital Général de Montréal. Their debts were so great that they had to resort to all sorts of new fund-raising activities, including making military garments and tents, establishing a brewery and a tobacco plant, and operating a freight and cartage business. Patients who regained health as a result of the nuns' charitable efforts were put to work to aid in the fund-raising effort (Gibbon and Mathewson, 1947, p. 47).

When war broke out between the British and the French in 1756, a section of the hospital called the Ward of the English was opened to care for the wounded English soldiers. The sisters were sufficiently generous of spirit to provide refuge to escaped English soldiers fleeing from the Indians. ". . . one of these English showed his gratitude, in 1760, by saving the hospital from the artillery fire of the army of invasion" (Gibbon and Mathewson, 1947, p. 48). In 1760 the transfer of authority over Montreal to the British brought with it statements testifying to the respect in which the sisters were held. General Amherst stated:

> Of the goodwill I have to a Society so worthy of respect as that of the Monastery of St. Joseph de l'Hôtel Dieu de Montréal, which can count so far as the British Nation is concerned on the same protection that it has enjoyed under French rule (Gibbon and Mathewson, 1947, p. 48).

Although French nursing orders extended invitations of welcome to the Canadian sisters after the war and a Canadian philanthropist offered to pay all expenses of the voyage, only two sisters accepted the offer. Most were thoroughly Canadian by now and did not wish to leave. However, abject poverty ensued after the war when communication became difficult with the wealthy citizens in France who had provided donations during the war. The sisters remaining in Canada became dependent on charity for some time.

There were striking differences between nursing in Britain and nursing in France in the 17th century, and these differences are fundamental to the quality of nursing in Canada in a historical context. Following the dissolution of the monasteries by Henry VIII subsequent to his renunciation of the Catholic church, the quality of nursing in England deteriorated when the nursing sisterhoods that had staffed the large London hospitals were ejected and the care fell into the hands of poorly qualified and unsuitable persons. Gibbon and Mathewson (1947) have observed that:

> If the Settlements along the St. Lawrence River had been colonized in the seventeenth century by the English instead of by the French, the history of nursing in Canada might have been very different. Fate, however, decided in favour of the French, and that was fortunate both for the Huron and Algonquin Indians and for the white pioneers, since in the wake of the fur traders and *coureurs de bois*, came the Augustinian Hospitallers or Nursing Sisters of Dieppe to Quebec and the St. Joseph Hospitallers of La Flèche to Montreal on their missions of healing and mercy, missions which had no counterpart in the colonizing efforts of the Protestant English in North America (p. 1).

It was the deterioration of nursing in England beginning in the 16th century that required the reforming efforts of Florence Nightingale some 3 centuries later. Nightingale incorporated fundamental ideas and approaches from the work of the nursing sisterhoods in Germany and in France.

Although there was a strict approach to ensuring cleanliness in the hospital, the concept of isolating those with infectious disease to prevent the spread of infection was still largely unknown. However, it was known that conditions under which animals were slaughtered for human consumption had to be healthy, and there is evidence in New France that meat inspection was carried out for this purpose. Heagerty quotes an edict issued in 1707 pertaining to the sale of meat:

> No butcher, under pain of confiscation and fine, may kill an animal without informing the King's Officer appointed for the purpose, or his representative, and bringing him to the place to ascertain if the animal was in a healthy enough state for public distribution of the meat. No inhabitant of the country may bring and sell meat in the town without presenting to the King's Officer or his representative a certificate from a judge, if there be one in the place of residence, or, if not, the seigneur, curé or military officer, which certificate shall state that the animals brought by them are not suffering from disease of any kind be-

fore being killed and that they did not die of accident, as for example, drowning or poisoning (Heagerty, 1980, p. 139).

Following the battle between the English and the French for the control of the territory of New France, the population received a large influx of United Empire Loyalists who left the United States as a result of the American War of Independence. It is estimated that 50,000 settlers came north, a large number settling in Nova Scotia and others moving further to settle along the St. Lawrence River and around the Great Lakes. Immigration from Britain began and large numbers of immigrants came over. However, many never made it to Canada as a result of rampant infectious disease due to unsanitary conditions on the old sailing ships. Others spread disease after their arrival. Following the arrival of a large number of Irish immigrants seeking to escape the potato famine, an epidemic of cholera wiped out ½ of the population of Montreal in 1832 (Hastings and Mosley, 1980). Because of such problems, efforts were made to prevent immigrants from spreading infectious diseases among the resident population, and a quarantine station was established at Grosse Isle in the St. Lawrence River. Arriving immigrants were required to stay to either recover from disease or demonstrate that they were free of it, and thousands and thousands of immigrants from Britain are buried at Grosse Isle. Although the idea of quarantine had considerable merit, it was found to be very difficult, if not impossible to ensure that all ships unloaded their passengers at Grosse Isle. Ships were able to allow passengers to disembark at a variety of locations along the River, and thus the quarantine was unsuccessful because it was almost impossible to enforce. If even one infected immigrant spread an infectious disease in the colony, it tended to negate all of the efforts to quarantine incoming settlers.

■ An Emerging Concept of Public Health

The origins of the public health movement in the last quarter of the 18th century can be attributed to recognition of the fact that the devastating epidemics that had ravaged society throughout the ages were caused by diseases resulting from the invasion of the body by specific organisms, the spread of which could be controlled by proper hygiene and other preventive measures. Although Jenner had discovered a vaccine that could prevent the development of smallpox in exposed individuals in 1796, the significance of his discovery in terms of the use of smallpox vaccination to prevent the disease in the population as a whole did not occur for a considerable length of time. It took well over a century for smallpox vaccination to become widespread practice and until the 1970s for the declaration of the eradication of the disease by the World Health Organization. Heagerty has pointed out that the phrase "public health" had not even been coined at the time of Confederation. Public thinking had not yet made the transition to the need for measures of control and care at the community level and was still focused on individual rather than public responsibility for health. The very fact that in passing the British North America Act of 1867, the fathers of Confederation vested primary responsibility for health in the provinces provides evidence that health was not thought to be sufficiently important or meaningful to be retained as a federal area of responsibility. Social consciousness about public responsibility versus private responsibility for health care and for promotion of health and prevention of disease has developed over the period since Confederation and the public-private debate relative to health care continues to be controversial to this day.

With the gradual recognition that the devastating impact of epidemic diseases could be reduced if not eliminated by measures of control involving the individual as well as the community, the case for developing measures to ensure that the community assumed responsibility for certain aspects of health promotion and care was strengthened. Nevertheless, the progression to social responsibility for health was hesitant and extended over a considerable period of time. Dawson and Younge noted that "The establishment of health and hospital services was essentially a 20th century development. Until the late 19th century, illness was everywhere considered an individual or family responsibility" (Dawson and Younge, 1940, p. 244). In such matters government intervention was seen as intrusive.

The scientific revolution in medicine and health began with the important discoveries by Semmelweiss and Lister. These discoveries, along with Pasteur's startling breakthrough rendering milk supplies safe through a process of heating, led to the introduction of asepsis in hospitals, pasteurization of milk, treatment of water supplies, and control of food. In addition the use of available vaccines to prevent disease became more common. However, the discovery of new knowledge is one thing and the institution of practices based on it quite another. To make their way into the public domain, public support for new practices is required, as well as a social consciousness about health. A great deal of work would be needed to ensure that people became more knowledgeable about the need to preserve and protect health so that they would be inclined to support community measures that could enhance these objectives.

Successive epidemics of cholera, diphtheria, scarlet fever, smallpox, tuberculosis, typhoid, and typhus led to the establishment of emergency committees or boards of health to develop community strategies to combat infectious disease. At the outset these tended to be temporary measures that saw the dissolution of the board after the epidemic subsided and the immediate threat was over. However, this represented community action for the purpose of controlling the epidemic. As noted by Heagerty (1980):

> There was no continuity of effort and nothing of a permanent nature in the way of sanitary measures. The average death rate was thirty-seven per thousand of the population, and during times of epidemic it ran as high as fifty or more per thousand, such as in the year 1885 when smallpox was epidemic in Montreal (p. 142).

The passage of a Public Health Act in Britain in 1875 provided a model for the colonies, and in 1884 Ontario passed public health legislation establishing a provincial board of Health (Hastings and Mosley, 1980). Quebec followed with a Public Health Act in 1886, spurred on by the impact of the epidemic of smallpox the previous year (Heagerty, 1980). The provincial public health acts directed municipalities to appoint local boards of health, a medical officer of health and a sanitary inspector (Hastings and Mosley, 1980). Although from the time that provincial statutes began to appear the federal government received considerable pressure to establish a department of health, it would not do so until the public health movement gained greater strength. A federal Department of Health was thus established in 1919, and a Dominion Council of Health was announced at the same time and placed under its jurisdiction. The membership of the Council included the chief medical officer of each of the provinces and 5 lay members representing labour, agriculture, rural and urban women's organizations, and a scientific adviser (Heagerty, 1980). The development of voluntary organizations to support public health has also been identified as influencing public opinion and stimulating the development of public health legislation. As early as 1875, a citizen's public health association was formed in Montreal where the annual mortality rate was 34 per 1000 (Heagerty, 1980). Many other such organizations would follow as it became recognized that public support for the implementation of public health measures to prevent and control disease was necessary. Other important factors were the development of an educational system open to all, growing prosperity, the European immigration, application of democratic principles in all areas of life, better communication and transportation, and entrenchment of the idea of caring for and about others.

■ Public Health Nursing in the Modern Context

The reform of nursing and the development of the profession as a suitable occupation for lay women can be attributed to Florence Nightingale's work in the Crimea and Britain. Although Nightingale did not subscribe to the germ theory, she nevertheless advocated strict cleanliness and extended this to the patient and the environment. Her approach was one with a preventive as well as a curative thrust, since she spoke of nursing the well, as well as the sick. According to Nightingale, the aim of nursing should be to treat the patient in such a way as to allow the reparative processes of nature to act in the best possible way (Nightingale, 1859). By implementing high personal and professional standards for nurses, nursing practice based on the best available knowledge and respect for a patient as a person, Nightingale revolutionized nursing and patient care and served as a catalyst for public opinion on these matters.

The development of schools of nursing in Canada occurred after the worldwide publicity given to Nightingale's work and the establishment of her School of Nursing in association with St. Thomas' Hospital in London. The movement to establish schools of nursing along with the development of the early hospitals in the country was a parallel development to the emerging concept of public health. Because it was generally believed that those providing care on a 24-hour basis in the new hospitals should have appropriate knowledge and skills, the creation of schools went hand in hand with establishment of these health care institutions. The first school known as the Mack School after its founder, Dr. Theophilus Mack, was established in association with the General and Marine Hospital in St. Catharines, Ontario. Schools followed at Montreal General Hospital and at Toronto General Hospital and elsewhere in the late 1800s and into the early 1900s and often appeared in tandem with the founding of hospitals. Until the late 1930s and early 1940s, graduate nurses were not able to seek employment in the institutions where they had been educated, for the hospitals were staffed almost exclusively with student labour at a much lower cost than graduate staff. Graduate nurses were engaged primarily in private duty nursing where they were employed by individuals and families to provide nursing care to the sick in their homes. In the era preceding the widespread acknowledgment of the hospital as the appropriate locus of care because of its increasing technology and expert personnel, nurses were independent entrepreneurs and functioned primarily in community settings. However, schools of nursing, hospitals, and professionals struggled to survive through the 1930s in the face of widespread economic crisis. The social upheaval that resulted would stimulate both the development of a new health care structure and new roles for nurses both in hospitals and in the community.

After World War I when the League of Red Cross Societies encouraged its member nations to facilitate the cause of public health worldwide, the Canadian Red Cross Society developed a peacetime program that would have substantial impact on the health of people. According to Hastings and Mosley (1980):

> ... public health attention extended from the purely environmental aspects of community health control to include school health services and maternal and child health services. Stress was laid on education about measures for personal health and hygiene, as well as on the provision of special protection through immunization procedures. These developments led to the creation of a new public health worker, the public health nurse (pp. 149-50).

Nurses became front-line personnel in the community for the promotion and maintenance of health and for the prevention and control of disease. Nursing responsibilities extended to screening programs to detect disease at an early stage, to activities to assist in maintaining a healthy environment, and to offering personal nursing services. From the outset, the development of programs to prevent disease and promote health became the responsibility of the official agency operated by municipal and provincial governments further to provisions of programs identified in public health acts. Voluntary organizations such as the Canadian Red Cross Society and the Victorian Order of Nurses developed programs on a national level which involved visiting nursing, health education and in some cases the operation of small cottage hospitals.

One of the objectives of the Canadian Red Cross Society in its postwar thrust to promote public health was to prepare nurses for public health work. Grants were given to universities across the country in 1920 to develop courses in public health nursing. Six universities across the country received funds to initiate the development of public health nursing courses. The universities that received funds included the University of British Columbia, the University of Alberta, the University of Western Ontario, the University of Toronto, McGill University, and Dalhousie University. The duration of the grants program was 3 years from 1920 to 1923, after which time the universities in question were expected to absorb the programs within their own budgets. With one exception, all of the programs in the 6 institutions were continued by the respective universities and eventually developed into degree programs. The University of British Columbia had been the first Canadian institution to initiate a degree program in nursing, just prior to the Red Cross grants (Zilm and Warbinek, 1994). Thus public health served as the catalyst for the development for university nursing education in Canada and it has continued over the years as a primary thrust in degree programs. A movement to restructure university nursing programs developed following Kathleen Russell's experimentation in curriculum design and the subsequent implementation of a basic integrated degree program in nursing at the University of Toronto in 1942. The release of the *Report of the Royal Commission on Health Services in 1964* castigating universities for perpetuating the 5-year nonintegrated programs in nursing sounded the bell for change in university nursing programs. However, as these sweeping changes in programs were implemented, public health would remain as a prominent area of study in the new curricula that emerged (Allemang, 1995).

Visiting Nursing

In the late 1890s, Lady Ishbell Aberdeen, wife of the Governor-General of Canada, became convinced of a need for better health services on the part of people all over the country. She and her husband had done a great deal of travelling and she saw the needs of the women because of a lack of facilities for childbirth and for health services by other isolated groups of people. Lady Aberdeen's idea was to develop an order of visiting nurses modelled after the Queen's Nurses in Britain to provide visiting nurses for people in their homes and in little cottage hospitals. Her plan had the support of women's groups all over the country but was blocked at first by physicians who stated that standards of care would be lowered and that nurses were unqualified to give the kind of care that was needed. Finally, Lady Aberdeen enlisted the assistance of Dr. Alfred Worcester, a noted Professor of Hygiene at Harvard, to come to Ontario to speak to Ontario physicians about the value of the plan. Subsequently a plan to establish the Victorian Order of Nurses (VON) was approved and Charlotte MacLeod from New Brunswick was appointed as the first Superintendent of the VON. The first VON nurses were pioneers in the true sense of the word. They were posted to remote locations across the country where they had to cope with life on the frontier. The first four nurses were posted to Fort Selkirk with a military detachment in 1898 during the Klondike Gold Rush. The VON continued to grow and flourish as these nurses met health needs in all parts of the country and, in particular, remote locations. The VON provided bursaries for study in public health nursing from 1921 onwards. There was a return in service commitment to the VON, and many nurses continued with the VON after their commitment had been fulfilled following graduation.

VON programs were planned according to the needs in a particular community and included both preventive and restorative approaches to meeting the health needs of their clients. The innovative approach of the VON and their ability to transfer responsibility for services to other agencies as this seemed desirable or necessary has characterized the way in which they have functioned across the country. In many urban and rural areas, the VON was the sole provider of visiting nursing services for decades. Even though more recently, responsibility for the provision of publicly-funded home health services has tended to be assumed entirely by the municipal departments of health in many areas of the country, VON branches continue to operate and to provide a variety of needed community nursing and other health services. It seems reasonable to suggest that the success of the VON was linked to its adaptability and its ability to offer relevant and needed services to the population.

There were variations in the visiting nursing model that developed across the country. For example, in Alberta, what was known as district nursing developed on the British model. Midwifery was a primary area of practice of these nurses who were first appointed in 1919. The isolated conditions under which a great many women lived on the frontier required the development of a number of approaches to providing assistance for them. District nursing was one such approach. The development of the Certificate Program in Advanced Practical Obstetrics at the University of Alberta in 1942 was directly related to the educational needs of district nurses who were allowed to practice midwifery under legislation that specified the conditions under which these nurses were able to practise in northern and isolated areas of the province.

The systematic neglect of the roles played by nurses in documented histories of health care organizations is evident in local histories of hospitals and health agencies. This reflects values prevalent in society over time and is not unique to the health field. However, the greater prominence given in historical records to work performed by men over that of women seems curiously inappropriate when viewed through the lens of contemporary standards. Clearly there is a relationship here to nursing as a profession that has historically attracted women to its ranks. With a few notable exceptions, many of the histories of health care organizations consist of little more than biographical sketches of physicians associated with the organization over time with little or no mention of other individuals and groups contributing to the growth and development of the institution. Given the primary roles fulfilled by nurses in nearly all of these organizations, the omission of discussion of their work is striking. The status accorded physicians in the histories of organizations would seem to parallel their status in the health care field. As Stuart has pointed out, "By 1900, physicians had ensured their control over hospitals, and were sending their patients there. They also moved to dominate the field of public health." (p. 53). In doing so they became the superiors of nurses and policy decisions were vested in their realm of responsibility. The manner in which gender conflict in public health in the 1920s was evident, and approaches that public health nurses in Ontario took to cope with it have been explored in some detail by Stuart. She points out that public health nurses who participated in the Ontario Provincial Board of Health's child welfare demonstration project of the 1920s shouldered an enormous amount of responsibility for the success or failure of the project. These nurses practised hundreds of miles from the nearest physician and took the place of physicians where necessary. Thus Stuart concluded that these circumstances "precluded a passive and subordinate stance." (p. 50).

Although the undervaluing of women's work has undoubtedly contributed to a dearth of literature about public health nurses and nursing, it may also have been a factor in their relatively low profile in public health work and indeed the invisibility of nursing and nurses even though nurses were the front line professionals who carried out public health programs at the community level in health agencies. There are other barriers to documenting and discussing the role and contributions of nurses in public health and some of the factors referred to may well have influenced these as well. Lack of records and other sources of primary information about health department operations and in particular the work of public health nurses are an example of a serious problem for those who attempt to pursue historical questions of interest pertaining to public health and public health nursing. Even though histories of organizations and exploration of historical questions of professional work are undertaken by a variety of writers, the level of understanding of the mission of the organization and the work performed by its professional nurses has been seen to be critical to an objective and balanced portrayal of the organization.

In conclusion, public health nursing clearly grew out of the charitable and philanthropic work of middle and upper class women with the sick poor in the community. As public health nursing became identified as a unique and specialized area of nursing, women's groups championed its legitimacy and stood up to opposition of the medical profession on the one hand and to political parties on the other to support the development of public health nursing services. The services of public health nurses were seen as vital to the health of the community in a society which was repeatedly devastated by epidemics of a variety of infectious diseases for which there were no effective treatments. Prevention through immunization and health education became accepted as the most useful approach to preventing the spread of infectious diseases and public health nurses were seen as the front-line professionals who could most successfully carry out public health programs targeted to these objectives. Nurses employed to carry out public health responsibilities have carried out their responsibilities with distinction over a lengthy period of time. As the community is emerging in the present context as the setting in which both curative and preventive services will be offered in the future, the challenges are new and some may say that they are perhaps even greater than they have been in the past.

■ REFERENCES

Allemang, M.M. (1995). Development of community health nursing in Canada. In M.J. Stewart (Ed), *Community nursing: Promoting canadians' health.* Toronto: W.B. Saunders.

Boutilier, B. (1994). Helpers or heroines? The National Council of Women, Nursing, and "Woman's Work" in late Victorian Canada. In D. Dodd & D. Gorham (Eds.), *Caring and curing: Historical perspectives on women and healing in Canada* (pp. 17-48). Ottawa: University of Ottawa Press.

Brown, G. (Ed.). (1966). *Dictionary of Canadian biography: 1000 to 1700* (vol. 1). Toronto: University of Toronto Press.

Canadian Red Cross Society. (1962). *The Canadian Red Cross Society: The role of one voluntary organization in Canada's health services—A brief to the Royal Commission on Health Services.* Toronto: The Society.

Dawson, C.A. & Younge, E.R. (1940). *Pioneering in the prairie provinces: The social side of the settlement process.* Toronto:

Gibbon, J.M. & Mathewson, M.S. (1947). *Three centuries of Canadian nursing.* Toronto: The Macmillan Co.

Hastings, J.E.F. & Mosley, W. (1980). Introduction: The evolution of organized community health services in Canada. In C. Meilicke & J. Storch (Eds.), *Perspectives on Canadian health and social services policy: History and emerging trends* (pp. 145-155). Ann Arbor, MI: Health Administration Press.

Heagerty, J.J. (1980). The development of public health in Canada. In C. Meilicke & J. Storch (Eds.), *Perspectives on Canadian health and social services policy: History and emerging trends* (pp. 137-144). Ann Arbor, MI: Health Administration Press.

Jamieson, E., Sewall, M., & Gjertson, L. (1959). *Trends in nursing history.* Philadelphia: W.B. Saunders.

Juchereau, J.F. & Duplessis, M.A. (1959). *Trends in nursing history.* Philadelphia: W.B. Saunders.

Kenton, E. (1925). *The Jesuit relations and allied documents.* New York: The Vangard Press.

Miller, G. (Ed.). (1983). *Letters of Edward Jenner and other documents concerning the early history of vaccination.* Baltimore, MD: Johns Hopkins University Press.

Millman, M.B. (1965). In G. Griffin & J. Griffin (Eds.), *Jensen's history and trends of professional nursing* (pp. 423-439). St. Louis: Mosby-Year Book.

Nightingale, F. (1858). *Notes on nursing: What it is and what it is not.* London: Harrison.

Parkman, F. (1897). *The Jesuits in North America in the seventeenth century.* Boston: Little, Brown & Company.

Stuart, M. (1994). Shifting professional boundaries: Gender conflict in public health, 1920-1925. In D. Dodd & D. Graham (Eds.), *Caring and curing: Historical perspectives on women and healing in Canada* (pp. 49-70). Ottawa: University of Ottawa Press.

Thwaites, R.G. (1959). *The Jesuit relations and allied documents: Trends and explorations of the Jesuit missionaries in New France (Vols I to XII).* New York: Pageant Book Company.

Zilm, G. & Warbinek, E. (1994). *Legacy: History of nursing education at the University of British Columbia 1919-1994.* Vancouver: University of British Columbia School of Nursing.

2 The Shape and Structure of Health Care in Canada

Janet Ross Kerr

The importance of health-care financing to society is reflected in the nature and quality of the service available, eligibility for and access to health care, and the affordability and accountability of the system. For health care professionals, the very essence of their practice depends on the way in which the system is financed. In the case of nurses, the fact that they are primarily employees of health-care agencies means that as the quantity of health care available in a publicly funded system is alternately expanded and withdrawn as a result of economic and political forces, the opportunity to practise is also subject to the uncertainties of resource allocation. The relevance of this situation is that every professional group needs to fully understand and actively participate in the debate over financing arrangements. No subject is more controversial and none is more vital than the nature and types of services to be provided, identification of which professional or occupational groups will provide them, determination of whether health care will be funded from public or private sources, and the form of remuneration for each group providing health care. Nurses need to be conversant with the issues in health-care financing and to participate actively in the discussion and determination of how these issues will be resolved both in their professional groups and as individuals (Ross Kerr, 1996).

■ Constitutional Responsibility for Health

The value placed on life in contemporary society is reflected in arrangements to promote good health in the population and provide health care for those who require it. Under the terms of The British North America Act of 1867, responsibility for health was given to the provinces, a division of powers maintained in The Constitution Act of 1982. When the founding fathers decided to make health a provincial mandate, times were very different and health was not a priority of the fledgling colonial government. Since the era of remarkable scientific discoveries and concomitant advances in health knowledge had not yet commenced, the importance of health in the ensuing century and beyond would have been difficult to envision. The emergence of Canada as a progressive nation through nurturing of its social democratic traditions from the colonial era through the transition to full and independent partnership in the Commonwealth had major implications for societal perceptions of the necessity to offer health care on a just and equitable basis to all citizens.

■ The Evolution of Medicare

The initial attempts to develop prepaid medical and hospital insurance were born of war, depression, and social upheaval. The original plan for prepaid health care began "... in the early years of World War I when rural municipalities in Saskatchewan began to employ physicians on contract to provide general practitioner services through local property taxes and 'premiums' for non-property owners" (Taylor, 1980, p. 184). Plans to prepay hospital services developed in conjunction with the municipal doctor program and "by 1939, about 100 municipal plans were operating" in Saskatchewan (p. 184). The heartbreaking suffering of people who could not afford health care gave leaders such as Premier Tommy Douglas in Saskatchewan the conviction and the motivation to work for conditions under which health care would be a service paid for through the system of taxation. As a child, Douglas had suffered from osteomyelitis in one of his legs. The standard treatment of the day was amputation, but Douglas was identified from his standard ward hospital bed as an interesting candidate for a new procedure to remove the infected part of the bone by a visiting private surgeon. He was given the opportunity to have the surgery, however, not because he was deserving, but because the demonstration of the procedure was seen as important for the teaching of medical students. Thus, instead of going through life as an amputee, Tommy Douglas was given a new lease on life, and he went on to become a middle weight boxing champion and later, Premier of Saskatchewan. Douglas' own experience was clearly influential in shaping his thinking about the structure and financing of health care. He stated many years later in the legislature of Saskatchewan that he had made his commitment to equal access to health care at an early age. Advocating a national health insurance scheme required a fundamental shift in thinking about health care as a privilege to health care as a right and was as much a matter of controversy in the early decades of the 20th century as it is today. The fact the Saskatchewan became the first area of the country to pass legislation allowing municipalities to raise taxes to support the employment of physicians, the establishment of hospitals and the development of hospital and medical insurance plans is important because the province was perhaps the region of the country most deeply affected by the poverty accompanying the Depression. The experience with prepaid hospital and medical care in Saskatchewan provided the springboard for the passage of legislation in 1947 establishing the first compulsory hospital insurance plan in North America by the Cooperative Commonwealth Federation party, the party first elected 3 years before under Douglas' leadership. In the forefront of health-care financing in the country, the Saskatchewan model would influence the federal government to bring in a health-care financing package offering universal access to health care to all residents, which would include all provinces by 1971.

The National Health Grants Act of 1948

In 1945 the federal government had developed plans for a scheme of national health insurance, but despite positive public opinion, the federal offer was rejected by the wealthiest provinces and the initiative collapsed. Instead, in 1948, the last year of Prime Minister Mackenzie King's term in office, his Liberal government brought in the National Health Grants Act, legislation which provided financing for hospital construction and was comparable in many ways to the Hill-Burton Act in the United States. Because there had not been any progress federally, in 1949 British Columbia and Alberta developed their own compulsory hospital insurance plans. Also in 1949, Newfoundland with its publicly-administered cottage hospital system joined Confederation. Thus another province was committed to national health insurance. The ranks of the four provinces already committed to a national plan were augmented in 1955 by Ontario, which "joined these four in pressuring the federal government to honour at least the hospital benefit stage of its 1945 health insurance offer." (Taylor, 1980, p. 187). With a large proportion of the Canadian population in five provinces on board, the federal government at last had the mandate to move ahead with its proposals.

The Hospital Insurance and Diagnostic Services Act of 1957

Thus the passage of The Hospital Insurance and Diagnostic Services Act in 1957 offered federal assistance for "prepaid coverage universally available to all residents, including diagnostic services to in-hospital patients and a broad range of out-patient services" (Taylor, 1980, p. 189). The plan involved a 50-50 cost-sharing arrangement for in- and out-patient hospital services. Because of the constitutional power of the provinces relative to health, each province had the opportunity to decide whether or not to join in the national effort. However, because the plan involved 50-50 cost sharing, any province that chose not to join would forfeit its own tax dollars and effectively subsidize the plans operating in the other provinces to "go it alone." When the Act came into force in 1958, the five provinces that had expressed support for the national plan, agreed to participate. However, by 1961 all provinces had agreed to do so. Excepted from the national hospital insurance program were tuberculosis and mental hospitals and certain other health institutions. As a result of the implementation of this plan, Blue Cross plans and plans operated by other insurance companies phased out coverage for a standard ward hospital bed and shifted their focus to other hospital benefits that were not covered.

The Medical Care Insurance Act of 1966

Medical care was not a part of the health insurance coverage offered to the provinces in The Hospital Insurance and Diagnostic Services Act. Although the General Council of the Canadian Medical Association had passed a resolution in January, 1943 endorsing the principle of health insurance, with the expansion of the prepaid medical plans sponsored by the profession this policy was changed in the early 1950s (Taylor 1980, pp. 185, 187). Again, Saskatchewan was to be the catalyst in the transition to prepaid medical insurance available on a universal basis to residents of Canada. The Douglas government was quite aware of the fact that the development of prepaid hospital insurance was its most important legislative success, and it proceeded to extend this to cover physicians' services despite the vehement opposition of this powerful professional group. The ensuing physicians' strike in Saskatchewan was a bitter struggle that shocked the country and lasted 23 days. In the end there was compromise with the provincial government allowing physicians to opt out of the plan and bill patients directly if they chose to do so, and the physicians conceding "to the government the right to enrol everyone and to determine benefit levels" (Taylor, 1980, p. 188). This led to the federal Medical Care Insurance Act of 1966, which expanded the system of prepaid hospital coverage to include medical care for all residents of Canada. The controversial nature of the legislation may explain the participation of only two provinces at the time the legislation became effective on July 1, 1968. However, the federal government undoubtedly took some of its cues from the Saskatchewan experience and allowed a 5-year period of time for all provinces to enter into a federal-provincial arrangement for the prepayment of medical services. The plan covered physicians' services in and out of hospital but did not prevent provinces from allowing physicians to opt out of the plan. It also did not prevent them from billing patients directly, requiring them to seek reimbursement from the plan or imposing surcharges on the established fee for a particular service.

The Fiscal Arrangements and Established Programs Financing Act of 1977

Because health costs had escalated by the early 1970s and because health-care expenditures as a proportion of Gross Domestic Product were continuing to rise, the federal government was concerned about the open-ended or 'blank cheque' approach of the 50-50 cost sharing arrangement of the hospital insurance act. The passage of The Fiscal Arrangements and Established Programs Financing Act in 1977 replaced 50-50 cost sharing with block funding. The latter involved transfer of some tax points to the provinces and reduced the federal contribution to health care to 25%. Additional federal contributions were based on increases in Gross Domestic Product. Dissatisfied with the fee schedule negotiated between their professional group and the provincial government in the late 1970s, physicians were increasingly using copayments or extrabilling to ensure that fees for various services were as high as they believed they should be. There was also a similar concern about another form of copayment called user fees for various forms of institutional services.

The Canada Health Act of 1984

To address its concerns about the erosion of medicare, the federal government passed The Canada Health Act of 1984. Under its provisions, extrabilling and user fees were disallowed and a new clause was added to allow federal reimbursement for the services of "health practitioners" in addition to physicians and dental surgeons. This provision opened the door for nurse practitioners to be used to provide a broad range of primary health-care services, where funding for these had formerly been restricted to physicians. Although physicians were strongly opposed to the passage of legislation which would disallow extrabilling, the Act was passed by the Liberal government of Pierre Elliott Trudeau. A reflection of the enduring popularity of medicare is found in the fact that a new Progressive Conservative government elected in 1984 did not make any move to amend the legislation or to develop new proposals, even though it was 'lukewarm' to national health insurance.

Facility Fees and the Impending Loss of Federal Funding for Medicare

Elected in 1984, the Mulroney government downplayed the Canada Health Act during its 8 years in power by reducing federal contributions to provincial health-care plans and by allowing provinces to permit payment of "facility fees" by patients to physicians who performed surgical and other procedures in specially equipped suites and clinics in their offices. As the federal government turned a blind eye to the provisions of the Canada Health Act, physicians were permitted again to extrabill or charge the patient directly over and above what the provincial plan paid for physicians' services. The passage of an amendment to The Federal-Provincial Fiscal Arrangements Act and Federal Postsecondary Education and Health Contribution Act by the Progressive Conservative government of Prime Minister Brian Mulroney identified certain sequential targets for reducing and eventually eliminating deficit spending. It would have had the effect of reducing federal government contributions to health care on a rigid schedule until the federal share was eliminated entirely. At this point, The Canada Health Act would no longer carry any weight with the provinces because of the federal government's lack of jurisdiction over health care under the Constitution. Any power wielded by the federal government in health care has been strictly dependent on its role in financing provincial health plans; the old adage "he who pays the piper calls the tune" applies here. The Liberal government of Jean Chrétien, elected in 1993, weighed its courses of action carefully in the first 2 years of its mandate and also passed an amendment to these two federal acts, which was assented to on 24 March, 1994. The effect of this amendment was to extend the timetable for the gradual reduction of federal contributions to the provinces for health to March 31, 1999. This piece of legislation was a disappointment to many because it did not appear to maintain a relatively high level of federal contributions to health care, therefore no longer ensuring that provincial plans upheld federal standards through financing provincial plans. It is clear that the integrity of The Canada Health Act is still under attack, and it remains to be seen whether the highly popular system of national health insurance will survive in Canada.

■ The Philosophical Basis of Medicare

National health insurance has always been a highly popular program of provincial and federal governments, and Canadians have come to believe passionately in their right to health care supported by a system of health insurance. However, a task force of the Canadian Bar Association examined whether or not Canadians have a legal right to health care, concluding that "there is no right to health care under the *Charter of Rights and Freedoms.*" The exception to this was the province of Quebec, which passed legislation articulating the right to health care within certain parameters and as such represents "an innovative and useful model" for other provinces to consider (Canadian Bar Association, 1994, p. 37). However, the Report went on to state that "Notwithstanding the above, there is a general expectation among the Canadian public that there is a right to health care. As a result, there is a gap between the lack of a right to health care and the expectation by the public" (Canadian Bar Association, 1994, p. 26).

At the basis of the development of the national health insurance system are the five basic principles of health care, from which standards for the legislation are derived. The first principle, *universality*, refers to coverage offered to the population as a whole rather than to selected population groups. Therefore coverage is extended to all qualified residents. The principle of *comprehensiveness* ensures that all medically necessary services included in the plan are covered. Although at the outset extra-billing and user fees were permitted, since the passage of The Canada Health Act of 1984, such charges may not be applied for services that are covered by the plan. *Accessibility* of health care may be the most difficult to assure, since Canada's population is relatively sparse and spread over a vast territory. Reasonable access to medically necessary services is seen as essential, despite geographic and transportation difficulties. *Portability* or coverage for residents of a province who require health services just after a move or during a visit to another province is assured in plans, although there have been some difficulties with differential fees between provinces and obtaining full reimbursement from the home province. *Public administration* or non-profit administration of services by an organization fiscally responsible to the provincial government is also required. In the refinements made to the legislation since 1957, fine-tuning of the standards based on the five principles with which the provincial plans must comply to receive federal funding has been evident.

The philosophic basis for the development of the Canadian system of national health insurance is rooted in humanitarian and social democratic traditions. In a society in which life is a deep and enduring value, the health of people becomes an issue of fundamental importance. Ensuring that access to needed care is available to the population as a whole, rather than only to those with enough money to buy the care they need, reflects valuing of equality of citizens and the framework of social justice underlying the health-care system. Factors such as Canada's status as a colonial nation and major social upheavals of war and depression were undoubtedly significant in leading to the system of health insurance that evolved. Such a system requires that taxes are assessed and pooled to provide health care to the population. Pursuit of the common good has led the electorate to support the collection of tax revenue earmarked for health care and managed by governments for the provision of health-care services.

From the outset, the Canadian system of national health insurance developed in a similar fashion to systems in other Western countries. The fact that the provincial plans insure hospital care and care by physicians has meant dominant roles for hospitals and physicians in the system. The fact that the number of hospital beds increased at a rate much higher than the rate of population increase until the 50-50 federal/provincial cost-sharing arrangement was ended is significant. Care centred in the home and community health services of various types were areas not eligible for federal cost-sharing in the initial legislation. The exclusion of community-based health services from federal financing encouraged physician-centred, in-hospital care during the first 35 years of health-care legislation in Canada (Ross Kerr, 1996). The high cost of in-hospital care and using physicians as "gatekeepers" to the health-care system in the absence of health outcomes that were significantly better than the other Western nations spending less on health care has led to a search for more effective and efficient lower-cost alternatives. The "Alma-Ata" agreement by countries who are members of the World Health Organization of "health for all by the year 2000," has challenged western nations to adopt a more community-focused approach and one in which there is meaningful community involvement and influence. Health-care reform has become a slogan now being heard across the country. Although this term means different things to different people, there are some fundamental assumptions that the health-care system of the future will look quite different than that of today. It is expected that community-based care will enhance and facilitate health maintenance, health promotion, and prevention of disease, balancing these with measures to restore health:

> Many believe that it will not be possible to sustain the current system without major modifications. Task forces and commissions in most provinces are looking at ways to shift the heavy focus on physician and institutional care to 'community based' alternatives and non-physician providers (Deber, Hastings, & Thompson, 1991, pp. 73-74).

■ Threats to Medicare

It is evident that threats to medicare are not new and show no signs of diminishing. The issues are complex, interdependent and consequential. One of the difficulties that has been central to health-care reform across the country is the fact that the provinces and the federal government have been running large deficits for a number of years. As a consequence of failure to balance budgets, provincial and federal debt levels are such that the interest costs of servicing the debt have mounted to the point where they are becoming insupportable. Appeals to voters to endorse drastic cuts in government spending and services to eliminate deficit financing and to pay down debt are increasingly being heard by a concerned populace. Because health care is one of the most costly areas of government spending, it is fast becoming the target of intense budget slashing efforts. However, there are concerns about planning when dollars are cut out of health budgets in the absence of an overall plan for making the system more efficient. Because of the concerns, there are inherent and serious risks for both the present and future. It is somewhat alarming to see major cuts in health-care spending without first identifying the values and principles of the system and then determining ways in which the system could function more effectively. Also of concern is the possibility that needed reforms with their associated efficiencies will not occur because of political pressure applied by groups with vested interests.

The needs of professional groups must be balanced by the needs of society. In the evolving health-care system in Canada, there is a need for collaboration between professional groups. Up to now, the system has been such that governments attempted to cater to the demands of particular groups, when this may not have been to the benefit of clients or to the system as a whole. Although it is difficult to achieve consensus on contentious issues between professional groups, boards, and the public at large, it will be important to work toward this and to ensure that the voices of all interested parties are heard and given due consideration in the continuing debate over the shape and structure of health care. Governments are elected to act in the best interests of the people as a whole. Medicare is a highly popular program, and it is clear that programs must change in significant ways to achieve efficiencies. At the same time, it is important to maintain the integrity of the system in terms of the provision of a high standard of care to Canadians based on the basic principles fundamental to The Canada Health Act.

Limits to Resources Available

Limits to growth in the postindustrial society are increasingly being recognized in all sectors of human activity. In the expansionist decades of the 1950s and 1960s, it was believed that no health-care expense was too much for the public purse to bear. From 1970 onward it has become clear that consumption of health care will continue to rise unless the system is rationalized and made more efficient. The discussion is tempered by the fact that despite skyrocketing expenses, the health status of the population has not been increasing at a corresponding rate. In fact, when Canada's health status is compared to other developed countries using recognized indices, there does not seem to have been a benefit to spending more than most of these other countries. Ways of helping the population as a whole to recognize and adopt healthy lifestyles will be an integral part of efforts to make the system more affordable by reducing the general impact and the high cost of preventable health problems. In rationalizing the system it is important to identify health goals in Canadian society and to fine tune the delivery system to support these. Limits to resources must be considered as part of the process of rationalizing the health-care system for the system of the future must be supportable and sustainable.

Misuse of the System

Health-care clients are often accused by professionals and politicians of misusing the system. This is tantamount to saying that the average person is expected to understand the nature of a particular problem being experienced, how it should be solved and the most appropriate professional provider to consult about the particular problem. These expectations are terribly high and perhaps unrealistic. The practice of using emergency rooms for minor ailments rather than seeing physicians in their offices, medicentre locations, or primary health centres is often singled out as an example of misuse of the system by consumers. While some consumers clearly realize that emergency room care is inappropriate for minor problems, there are others who do not recognize this. The fact that emergency rooms in hospitals are available and have been accessed for minor complaints no doubt serves as a means of reinforcing the use of this service in an inappropriate way.

The other important idea in considering misuse is the fallacy in the assumption that misuse is client-driven. It is important to recognize that in many cases use that can be termed misuse is provider-driven and routine, but unnecessary follow-up visits to physicians or directions by the physician to come to the emergency room where it is more convenient for the physician are examples of provider-generated misuse of the system. Roos (1992) has identified geographic areas where high rates of particular types of surgery can be mapped. These are clearly provider-generated and undoubtedly represent misuse of the system. Even annual physical examinations are being questioned as unnecessary and costly to the health-care system despite the fact that the population has been led to believe that these examinations are essential to health promotion and disease prevention. Whether or not it is possible to change the health behaviour of the population in forgoing yearly physical examinations is not known. However, if physicians and nurses are used differently and to better advantage in the system, much more than this may be possible.

Maldistribution of Physicians

The maldistribution of physicians across the country in the face of an oversupply of these highly trained professionals is widely recognized as a problem. However, few solutions have emerged in this continuing debate. Physicians have historically been reluctant to locate their practices in areas remote from large urban centres. This is also true of other health professionals, but the independence of physicians with their private practices means that they have more control over where they will live and work. Because physicians are reimbursed for their services on a fee-for-service basis subject to terms and conditions placed on the fee schedule under provincial health plans, there have been efforts by provincial governments to try to influence where physicians practice by a number of means. This has been challenged in a lawsuit in British Columbia after the province implemented a system of assigning billing numbers for the number of physicians deemed necessary for each location in the province, thus limiting the number of physicians who could bill the health-care plan for services and therefore the supply of physicians. The Supreme Court of Canada upheld the physicians' side of the dispute and the province was no longer allowed to match billing numbers with needs of communities, thereby restricting the supply of physicians. Since then, measures have been instituted in some provinces to control costs, such as capping the total amount available for medical services, limiting overall amounts physicians are allowed to bill the plan annually and limiting the number of physicians who can move to a province and bill the plan for services. Discussions about changing the method of remunerating physicians from fee-for-service to salary or contract are occurring on a widespread basis. As provinces move to implement regionalization of health services in a continuing quest for a more efficient and effective health-care system, a more cost effective means of expending funds for physicians' services is likely to be high on the agenda.

Underutilization of Nurses

Nurses have historically been underutilized in the health-care system. This has resulted in part from the entrenchment of medicare beginning with legislation to provide funds for hospital construction in 1948 and continuing with hospital insurance legislation passed in 1957 and the prepaid medical insurance legislation of 1966. Physicians and hospitals have been dominant in health insurance legislation and this has injected an acute care and in-patient hospital focus to the approach to health care over the more than 40 years of federal financing of health care in Canada. From roles as private entrepreneurs in the early part of the century, nurses became employees in the health-care agencies which evolved after widespread unemployment during the Depression, while physicians continued to be private entrepreneurs, able to control the nature and extent of their practices as well as the location in which they provided their services. Although nurses were employed largely by hospitals in the

30-year period after World War II, the tremendous expansion in the number and size of hospitals resulted in a corresponding increase in the number of positions for registered nurses, even though nursing auxiliaries increasingly were employed in hospitals. In addition to the increased demand for nurses, their roles have continually expanded in almost all areas of practice and especially in a variety of areas of specialized practice as a result of the burgeoning increases in technology and in health knowledge.

Nursing education entered the university after World War I when the demand for nurses with public health knowledge was first heard. From certificate programs in public health nursing, universities eventually developed undergraduate degree programs in nursing incorporating a basic generalist knowledge of nursing including public health and health assessment. Graduate programs at the master's level followed in the post war expansionary period and concentrated on developing skills in advanced nursing practice and research. Doctoral programs in nursing have been established recently and have extended the range of preparation available in nursing. Nursing education has been becoming more sophisticated over the past two decades with increased numbers of baccalaureate and master's degree students and a greater proportion of students entering initial programs of nursing education being admitted to programs offering a baccalaureate degree in nursing. Master's degree programs are available in all areas of the country and admit greater numbers of students, while the five doctoral programs in nursing are concentrated in British Columbia, Alberta, Ontario, and Quebec. In some provinces, the percentage of registered nurses prepared at the baccalaureate level is over 20%, and this figure is rising quickly.

It is evident that nurses are and have been receiving sophisticated preparation to meet the needs of a changing health-care system. However, it is still evident that their skills are not being used to greatest advantage because of the entrenchment of the physician and hospital domination of health care. In an environment where all of the assumptions upon which service delivery is based are being questioned, it is likely that nurses will be increasingly called on to use the full range of their skills to benefit the health-care consumer. As the focus of health care shifts to the community, nurses are in a unique position to serve the needs of clients because the degree programs in which more and more nurses have been prepared have always recognized the importance of community health nursing and have devoted a considerable amount of time to instruction in this area. It is likely that in the shift to the community, nurses who have been prepared in diploma programs will require further preparation in community health to allow them to make the transition to the health-care system of the future. More effective utilization of nurses will allow physicians to concentrate on areas of diagnosis and treatment that require their specialized expertise, and it is likely that improved health-care outcomes and a more efficient and effective system will result.

■ What Does the Future Hold?

The health-care system is likely to look very different in the future. The changes that are being rapidly imposed are extensive and wide-ranging, covering virtually all areas of health care. The system of the future will incorporate principles of primary health care to a much greater extent than the system that has been dominant to date in Canada. Consumers, who are considerably more knowledgeable today than their counterparts of yesteryear, will be much more informed and involved in decision making about their own health care. The efforts of health-care professionals will increasingly be directed towards educating consumers so that they can assume more responsibility for their own health. The community focus will mean the development of cost-efficient community health centres to which consumers may go for assistance with their health-care needs. The first health professional a consumer will see in a nonemergent situation, however, will likely be a nurse rather than a physician, since physicians will no longer be the "gatekeepers" to the system. Home visits by home-care nurses will be common as consumers cope at home with conditions and treatment for those conditions for which they would previously have been hospitalized. An integrated multidisciplinary focus will become a reality with all health professionals working together for the interests of the client, rather than in an isolated fashion in different locations in the community. Social and cultural determinants of health require much study and attention in order to produce improved health outcomes. The political framework within which the issues relative to health-care insurance plans are debated and determined will be conditioned by the economic and social realities of effecting fundamental change in the system. Decisions to move to a community-based model emphasizing prevention of disease, promotion of health and partnerships between professionals and consumers will be difficult ones but are those that will ultimately hold the greatest potential for impacting health positively. Issues surrounding hospital governance, education of health professionals, the integration of boards of health agencies on a regional basis, restructuring systems for providing care and for remunerating health professionals in a reasonable and rational way must be considered in a collaborative manner to allow the health-care system in Canada to meet the challenges which are ahead in this century and beyond. The opportunity for better, as well as less expensive, health care as a result of the shifting focus of care is there, and it remains to be seen whether the potential is realized.

■ References

Canadian Bar Association. (1994). *What's law got to do with it?* Ottawa: The Association.

Deber, R.B., Hastings, J.E.F., & Thompson, G.G. (1991). Health-care in Canada: Current trends and issues. *Journal of Public Health Policy, 12*(1), 72-82.

Roos, N.P. (1992). Hospitalization style of physicians in Manitoba: The disturbing lack of logic in medical practice. *Health Services Research, 27*(3), pp. 361-384.

Ross Kerr, J.C. (1996). The organization and financing of health care: Issues for nursing. In J.C. Ross Kerr & J. MacPhail (Eds.), *Canadian nursing: Issues and perspectives.* (pp. 216-227). Toronto: Mosby–Year Book.

Taylor, M.G. (1980). The Canadian health insurance program. In C.A. Meilicke & J.L. Storch (Eds.), *Perspectives on Canadian health and social services policy: History and emerging trends.* (pp. 181-219). Ann Arbor, MI: Health Administration Press.

3 Primary Health Care and the Health of Communities

JANNETTA MACPHAIL

Primary health care is purported by the World Health Organization (WHO) as the means for promoting and maintaining the health of nations around the world. What is the meaning of the concept of primary health care? Why is it endorsed and proclaimed as the solution to many ills in existing health-care systems? Is it a feasible goal for Canada? What reforms will be required in Canada's health-care system to implement the concept? Does the profession of nursing support the concept? Are nursing students being educated to function effectively in a primary health-care system? These questions are addressed as the meaning and significance of primary health care and the health of communities are explored.

■ Health for All By the Year 2000

The goal of Health for All by the Year 2000 was established in 1978 at an international meeting held at Alma-Ata in Kazakh Republic of the Soviet Union, under the auspices of WHO and the United Nations International Children's Emergency Fund (UNICEF) (WHO, 1978a). The meeting, attended by representatives of 127 nations and 72 international organizations, was to promote the concept of primary health care (PHC) as the only viable means of attaining equitable distribution of health resources to enable people to attain "a level of health that will permit them to lead a socially and economically productive life" (WHO, 1978b, p. 429). The report of the conference challenges all countries and governments of the world to employ a PHC approach with emphasis on the development of their health services. The approach is "based on practical, scientifically sound, and socially acceptable methods and technology made universally accessible to individuals and families in the community through their full participation and at a cost that the country can afford" (WHO, 1978b). The International Council of Nurses (ICN) pledged its full support to making PHC a reality in all countries of the world. Recognizing that most health care in the world is delivered by nursing personnel, ICN encouraged nurses in each country to participate in developing a PHC system that is relevant to the country's needs and uses nurses effectively in its implementation (WHO, 1978b, p. 429).

Commitment to the goal of Health for All by the Year 2000 led to another conference, held in Ottawa, Canada, in November 1986, which was organized jointly by WHO, Health and Welfare Canada, and the Canadian Public Health Association (CPHA). It was attended by 212 participants from 38 countries who met to exchange experiences, share knowledge, and develop a plan of action to achieve the goal. Those attending the meeting were representatives of a wide range of governmental, voluntary, and community organizations, as well as active practitioners and academics. The 3 main aims of the conference were to promote:

... *visibility:* to encourage and enhance health promotion development by assessing past and current achievements;

sharing: to put people in contact with each other, sharing examples of success and failure; and

consensus: to develop through the active participation of conference members a conference statement on the future development of health promotion (Nutbeam & Lawrence, 1987, p. 1).

The conference was primarily a response to growing expectations for a new public health movement around the world. It was built around 5 major issues, which participants discussed in workshops conducted over a 1-week period. The issues were building healthy public policy, creating supportive environments, strengthening community action, personal skills, and reorienting health services (Nutbeam & Lawrence, 1987). One outcome of the conference was the publication of the *Ottawa Charter for Health Promotion,* which identifies 3 elements basic to health promotion: advocating health, enabling people to achieve their fullest health potential, and mediating differing interests for the pursuit of health (Nutbeam & Lawrence, 1987).

The Honourable Jake Epp, Minister of National Health and Welfare Canada, chose the occasion of the conference to launch the Canadian government strategy document, *Achieving Health for All: A Framework for Health Promotion.* He emphasized that the purpose in releasing the document was to promote dialogue among Canadians interested in health and to achieve better health for ourselves and contribute to better health for the people of the world. His goal was to move health promotion from the periphery of the health field to a central position (Nutbeam & Lawrence, 1987).

■ The Canadian Approach to Achieving Health for All

The Canadian approach to achieving health for all is to focus on health promotion, which is perceived as the best strategy. Figure 3-1 identifies the overall aim, health challenges, health promotion mechanisms, and implementation strategies.

FRAMEWORK FOR HEALTH PROMOTION

AIM		Achieving health for all	
HEALTH CHALLENGES	Reducing inequities	Increasing prevention	Enhancing coping
HEALTH PROMOTIONS MECHANISMS	Self-care	Mutual aid	Healthy environment
IMPLEMENTATION STRATEGIES	Fostering public participation	Strengthening community health services	Co-ordinating healthy public policy

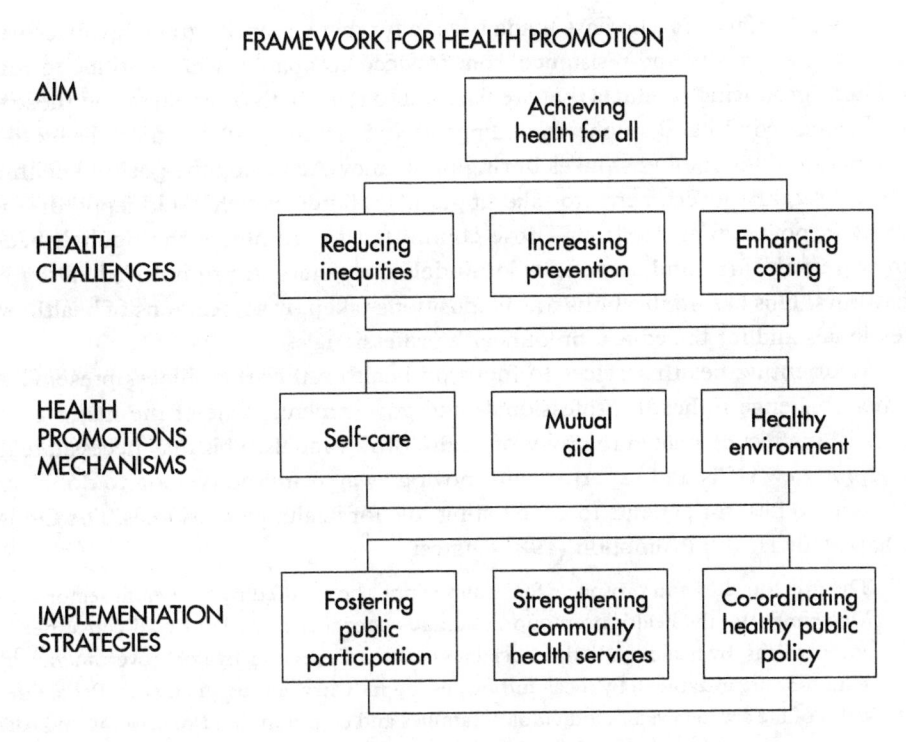

Figure 3-1 A framework for health promotion. (Modified from *Ottawa Charter for Health Promotion.* (1986). Ottawa: World Health Organization, Health and Welfare Canada, and the Canadian Public Health Association.)

Self-care, a mechanism supported by nurses, is defined in Epp's document as *the decisions and actions individuals take in the interest of their own health.* This concept supports nursing's goal of helping people to become increasingly responsible for their own health. However, creating conditions and surroundings conducive to health, which is implied in creating healthy environments, goes beyond the individual and requires community action. One example of this philosophy is creating a smoke-free environment, which cannot be accomplished by an individual; there must be agreement by groups, such as health-care institutions, businesses, and educational institutions. Considerable progress has been made in the past decade in attaining the goal of smoke-free environments as a result of community action, but the major public health problem of smoking is far from resolved.

Achieving healthy environments will require developing the political will "to overcome likely conflicts between public health interests and commercial and other vested interests" (Nutbeam & Lawrence, 1987, p. 2). This offers a real challenge to governments in relation to creating a smoke-free environment. They must provide alternatives for farmers who have made a living for many years by growing tobacco and deal with animosity and resistance from tobacco companies who continue to make millions producing products that are harmful to the health of smokers and those exposed to second-hand smoke, including the unborn fetus who is more likely to be premature if the mother smokes during pregnancy. Achieving the goal of health for all will require governments to take unpopular stands, which could jeopardize the party in power in an election. Those committed to promoting the public's health must remain firm and serve as role models for others in promoting healthy behaviours. This has implications for the positions taken by associations of health professionals and for the education of health professionals.

Reorienting health services to focus on health rather than illness presents another challenge to health professionals and governments. One of the major objectives is to effect change in the roles of health professionals. This may necessitate developing new skills and expertise and moving away from intervening to do what is considered best for patients to a mediating role for health professionals. The Ottawa Charter for Health Promotion (1986) states:

> The prerequisites and prospects for health cannot be ensured by the health sector alone. More importantly, health promotion demands coordinated action by all concerned: by governments, by health and other social and economic sectors, by non-governmental and voluntary organizations, by local authorities, by industry and by the media. People in all walks of life are involved as individuals, families and communities. Professional and social groups and health personnel have a major responsibility to mediate between differing interests in society for the pursuit of health (p. 1).

Government funding of health services in Canada continues to favour cure and sickness care strongly, with a minor proportion of the health-care dollar going to support health promotion and prevention of illness. Change in financial incentives are needed to support health promotion activities. Similarly, changes are needed in the initial and continuing education of health professionals to change their focus and priorities to primary health care and prepare them to help people achieve their fullest health potential and make decisions about matters that affect their health and well-being.

Maglacas, chief scientist for nursing with WHO, points out that although the aim of the Health for All movement has been interpreted by many as making health services available to everyone, the actual goal is to have all people in all countries achieve at least a level of health that allows them to work productively and participate actively in the social life of the community in which they live (CNA Connection, 1988). In 1987, almost 10 years after the WHO declaration at Alma-Ata, Maglacas (1988) assessed nursing's response to the Health for All challenge as "fragmented, sporadic, unplanned, and uncoordinated, and [as involving] few, if any, other disciplines or sectors" (p. 67). Primary health care, as envisioned by Maglacas and other nursing leaders, is perceived as the way to achieve the goal.

■ Primary Health Care

Primary health care (PHC) has been confused with primary medical care and primary nursing, but it is distinctly different from both. In the United States and in some parts of Canada, the concept of PHC is limited and tends to be equated with the nurse practitioner role. It is portrayed as a nurse, practising in an ambulatory setting or a remote site, who assesses the health and illness status of clients through "health history, physical examination, and diagnostic tests; develops and implements therapeutic plans; [and] engages in appropriate referrals, health counseling, and collaboration with other health care providers" (Ulin, 1982, p. 532). It is much like primary medical care and seems to be so when comparing nurse practitioner and physician practice in ambulatory care, such as reported by Diers, Hamman, and Molde (1986). Studies of nurse practitioner effectiveness, as compiled by Feldman, Ventura, and Crosby (1987) and as reviewed by Molde and Diers (1985), lend credence to this evaluation of the nurse practitioner role by Ulin.

Initial efforts to expand the role of the nurse in PHC in Canada followed the pattern of two types of practice, as identified by Allen (1977). The first type of practice is the assistant to the physician, which involves performing tasks delegated by the physician and is seen most commonly in physicians' offices and in family practice units. The second type is replacement of the physician, which signifies that the nurse performs the same tasks as the physician, although not those of the specialist, such as a surgeon. This type of practice is prevalent in remote areas in the north; in private practice, by nurses serving such populations as psychiatric patients; and in family practice units, where patients are allocated randomly to physicians and nurses depending on the availability of staff. Some nurses support the perspective of nurses replacing or substituting for physicians, as practised in the United States and carried out at McMaster University in the 1970s (Spitzer, Kergin, & Yoshida, 1975).

In 1972 the Boudreau Committee, which was established to address a gap in health-care services in Canada, recommended that short-term practitioner programs be developed in selected Canadian universities to prepare nurse practitioners to practise in remote sites, such as the far north, where physicians did not wish to reside and practise (Report of the Committee on Nurse Practitioners, 1972). Such programs were established, and all but one have been phased out. The remaining program is at Dalhousie University, which has continued because it includes a nurse-midwifery component that meets a need in outlying areas in the Atlantic region. The intent was to incorporate primary health-care concepts and physical assessment and history-taking skills into basic baccalaureate programs so that this essential content would be an integral part of the preparation of all nurses graduating from baccalaureate degree programs. This has been achieved, but the baccalaureate programs do not include preparation for the "physician substitute" skills that were included in some of the Canadian nurse practitioner programs to prepare them to practise in remote areas, where consultation was provided by physicians by telephone. Some of the nurse practitioners have practised in urban areas, usually in central city, under-served areas, where the poor, the unemployed, and the indigent seek health-care services from clinics. With the rapid expansion of knowledge and the knowledge base needed to make clinical decisions, it is recognized that short-term programs are not adequate to prepare nurses to practise in relatively independent, autonomous roles in which they actually substitute for physicians in remote areas.

The concept of primary health care envisaged by WHO is "essential health care made universally acceptable to individuals and families in the community by means acceptable to them, through their full participation and at a cost the community and country can afford" (Mahler, 1981, p. 5). The CNA views primary health care as "essential health care (promotive, preventive, curative, rehabilitative and supportive) that focuses on preventing illness and promoting health. [It] is both a philosophy of health care and an approach to providing health services [to] individuals, families, groups, communities and populations" (CNA, 1995, p. 1). Thus the concept is much broader than primary medical care and health promotion, although health promotion is the central focus, designed to enhance health potential and thereby maintain balance or stability. To achieve this goal "the focus in nursing must be moved to health and actions must move beyond the health sector and must involve the people themselves" (Maglacas, 1988, p. 67).

The key role for health professionals in this concept of primary health care is "empowering people to improve their lives and lifestyles, develop self-reliance and self-determination and take control of their health actions" (CNA Connection, 1988, p. 14). Fundamental changes in structure, roles, and relationships will be required to move from the present health-care system, which is increasingly expensive and emphasizes high technologies aimed at curing the few, to a very different and more widely available service built around health needs with individuals, families, and communities taking increased responsibility for their own health. The focus would be on community health and social centres in the community rather than a system centred in acute-care hospitals, for which 95% of the health-care dollar has been expended.

■ Nursing's Response to the Challenge

Are Canadian nurses and organized nursing in Canada prepared to support the changes needed to move to such a system of PHC? In the past decade the CNA has given high priority to considering the possibility and accepting the challenge. In September 1988, the CNA published a major document, *Health for All Canadians: A Call for Health Care Reform*, which provides an analysis of inadequacies in the existing health-care system and a vision of the changes needed and strategies to effect them to move to a system based on the philosophy and principles of PHC. The CNA envisions:

primary health care and its underlying principles of accessibility, public participation, health promotion, appropriate technology, and intersectoral cooperation [as] a natural extension of nursing practice, [and hence believes that] all nurses play a vital role in the implementation of primary health care (CNA, 1955, p. 1).

The CNA supports individuals, families, groups, and communities being active partners in their health care and recognizes the need for a major reorientation of health-care policies and health-care professionals to meet the challenges of the future.

In March 1989, the CNA board of directors approved a 5-year plan aimed at implementing this vision of PHC in Canada. It includes steps to define and clarify roles of nurses in PHC, to establish stable and adequate funding to facilitate demonstration projects, to examine the implications for educational programs in nursing, and to establish a lobbying campaign to expedite the development of PHC. "The major goals of the plan are to provide support for member associations to adopt and implement primary health care and to communicate the primary health care position at the national level" (CNA Connection, 1989). In March 1989, the CNA published a *Position Statement on the Nurses' Role in Primary Health Care*. Nurses are portrayed as having a key role that has 4 main aspects: "direct care provider; teacher and educator of health personnel and the public; supervisor and manager of primary health-care services; and researcher and evaluator of health care" (CNA, 1989). This was replaced by another statement in April 1995, which reflects progress, stating:

> The goal of nursing is to improve the health of clients through partnerships with clients, with other health care providers, related community agencies and government. Nursing practice involves a variety of roles including direct care provider, educator, administrator, consultant, policy advisor and researcher. The principles of primary health care apply to nurses in all these roles (CNA, 1995, p. 1).

Nursing already has a number of examples of their participation in PHC on which to build. Nurses practising in remote parts of Canada integrate principles of PHC, in varying degrees, in their daily practice (Chamberlain & Beckingham, 1987). In addition to the replacement model of practice seen in remote areas, Allen (1977) identified a complemental model. It differs from that of other health professionals, yet is complementary, so the client is provided with a more complete range of health-care services by experts. Allen developed such a model of practice in a "Health Workshop" staffed by faculty and students of the McGill University School of Nursing. The workshop, or health centre, was located in two middle-income, suburban communities, selected as representative of persons who consume large proportions of expensive medical services for lifestyle-related difficulties. They were also selected because existing models for improving health care were based largely on information from medically indigent populations and because families with young children tend to predominate in such suburban communities (Allen, 1981). The centre gave nurses the opportunity to help families "to examine their health habits and strategies for coping with life, practise new health behaviours, and search out healthy ways of living" (Warner, 1981, p. 34). The model was evaluated by Allen (1983), who reported that 83.2% of the persons brought health situations and 16.8% brought illness problems. "Approximately half the health contacts related to lifestyle and health behaviour, 20% to adaptation and management of illness, and 23% to changes in the family and interpersonal relationships combined" (p. 55). Although the model demonstrated that the health-care services provided were not available elsewhere and were needed, it did not continue because there was no mechanism for reimbursement of services through the existing health-care system. A need for change is indicated when a model that helped people become more self-reliant about their health and reduced the use of costly medical care services could not be supported and financed. Indeed, the model developed and tested by Allen applies most of the 5 principles of primary health care espoused today.

Increasing evidence suggests that alternative models for PHC are cost-effective and enhance the quality of care. For example, home visits by public health nurses in Ottawa resulted in greater mobility and higher morale among the elderly and fewer admissions to hospital (Flett, Last, & Lynch, 1980). In Manitoba, Ramsay, McKenzie, and Fish (1982) reported that patients who attended a clinic staffed by nurses achieved a greater decrease in blood pressure and greater weight loss than the patients attending a physician-staffed clinic. Similarly, persons in Newfoundland who received PHC delivered by nurses had a decrease in admissions to acute-care hospitals, whereas those receiving traditional physician-based care had a 39% increase in the use of acute-care hospitals (Denton, Gafini, Spencer & Stoddart, 1982). The length of hospital stay was shortened for patients who had members of the Victorian Order of Nurses (VON) involved in their discharge planning and follow-up care; and physical, social and emotional outcomes were improved for these patients, in comparison to patients who did not have VON nurses' care (Chambers & West, 1978). In a comparative study of the health behaviours of mothers in 3 primary-care settings in Quebec—a hospital clinic, a private physician's office, and a community health centre—nurses' care made a difference in the health behaviours of the mothers and the health status of children under 5 years of age (Thibaudeau & Reidy, 1977). Other examples have been cited in the literature, but they have not had a systematic evaluation component to assess outcomes. Hence there is need for designing and testing more primary health care models, in which nurses are the primary caregivers, and incorporating a sound evaluation component.

Approximately 40 government-funded community health centres have been developed in Ontario since 1973. It is estimated that there are also 160 in Quebec, 29 in the Atlantic provinces, and 35 in the prairie provinces and British Columbia. They use a multidisciplinary approach, employing a variety of health professionals, such as community, home care and palliative care nurses, nurse practitioners, nutritionists, physicians, physiotherapists and chiropodists, and nonprofessional staff to meet identified needs. Ontario's centres are reported to have reduced costs; the persons using them have had 16.7% fewer hospital days than those using the services of physicians in private practice. There is reported to be low turnover and increased accountability and commitment among nursing staff. While these centres are not the PHC model envisioned under nursing leadership, they have facilitated community outreach and provided opportunity for collaborative research, which is critical for health-care programming and evaluation (Innes, 1987).

The Association of Registered Nurses of Newfoundland (ARNN), in collaboration with the Danish Nurses Organization, have undertaken such a demonstration project. PHC is being practised by nurses in selected communities in Newfoundland, and outcomes are being evaluated in terms of measurable improvement in the health status of individuals and families and in health-directed lifestyles. The communities were involved in all aspects of program planning, implementation, and evaluation, which is an important concept in PHC. A major objective is to demonstrate that nurses can provide safe and effective PHC services in an affordable and cost-effective manner, and to develop a prototype of PHC that can be tested in other communities in Newfoundland, in other provinces, and worldwide (ARNN, 1987).

Because of concerns about the availability of PHC to the citizens of Alberta, the cost of health care, and the need for changes in the health-care system to fully utilize the potential of nurses, the Alberta Association of Registered Nurses (AARN) established a Task Force on Increased Direct Access to Nursing Services Provided by Registered Nurses in 1991. It included wide representation from consumers, government, other health-care providers, and nurses. "The AARN views increased direct access to registered nurses' services as a key component to successful, fundamental health care reform" (AARN, September 1993, p. 13). The challenge to the task force was to formulate strategies to increase direct access to nursing services in the community, and increase opportunities for remuneration of registered nurses through public funding. The outcome in 1993 was publication of a brochure and a booklet, both of which are entitled *Nurses: Key to Healthy Albertans,* to be used in educating the public, government, nurses and other health professionals. They contain basic aspects of the AARN proposal including the services that could be provided by nurses; the benefits of direct access in terms of health promotion and cost savings; and a recommendation to the Alberta government to fund nursing services that can be accessed directly by reallocating present health care funding from acute care to a community-based system. Examples of cost savings included are (1) a 1990 study that showed the cost of immunization by nurses in Alberta to be one-third the cost of immunization by physicians in Ontario (Sadoway, Plain, & Soskolne, 1990); (2) introduction of home-care services for low-birth-weight infants that resulted in an average savings of $18,000 per infant with no reduction in quality of care; (3) provision of home-care services through a community health centre employing nurses and volunteers resulted in 15% of clients choosing to be discharged from nursing homes and a 25% reduction in hospitalization (Jamieson, 1990); and (4) a 1979 study that showed the cost of home care for dying patients to be 25% less than hospital care (Kassakian, Bailey, Rinker, Stewart, & Yates, 1979). Moreover, there was evidence of improvement of quality of life for the subjects involved in these studies. To implement the goal of increased direct access to services provided by registered nurses, four targets have been identified: nurses, the public, government, and the AARN regions. An organized campaign is underway to maintain and increase support for the initiative, to increase the services provided by nurses in the community, and to make those services more visible to the public through the media and presentations within communities.

Rodger and Gallagher (1995) conducted a survey of the national/provincial/territorial nursing associations and community health nursing associations in Canada to determine strategies undertaken to support and apply the 5 principles of PHC: health promotion and illness prevention, accessibility to services, public participation, intersectoral and interdisciplinary collaboration, and appropriate technology. Responses were received from all 11 national/provincial nursing associations, from one of the two territorial associations, and from 7 of the 16 community health nursing organizations. Their findings revealed a variety of creative approaches to applying the principles, as well as resourcefulness and concerted efforts to support the goals of PHC in Canada. Many of the strategies focused on the principle of health promotion and illness prevention. For example, in addition to the Newfoundland-Denmark project by the ARNN cited previously, there are the Cheticamp PHC project undertaken by the Registered Nurses Association of Nova Scotia; health education programs in schools implemented by the Registered Nurses Association of British Columbia; a pilot project for a community-based health centre proposed by the Association of Nurses of Prince Edward Island; the Rankin Inlet Project undertaken by the Northwest Territories Registered Nurses Association to facilitate local birthing through the use of midwives rather than transport expectant mothers nearing term to southern health care facilities; and many health promotion projects in Quebec involving nurses in key roles. Most of these projects also address the principle of increasing accessibility to health care services. For the past decade the CNA and all provincial/territorial nursing associations have opposed strongly attempts to decrease accessibility through user fees and extra billing, which continue to present a threat with the drastic downsizing of health care resources in such provinces as Alberta. In addition, for many years the nursing organizations have endeavoured to increase accessibility through proper utilization of nurses as additional points of entry to the health care system.

Responses from the nursing organizations revealed nurses as strong proponents of the principle of public participation, as reflected in the investment of funds to prepare public service announcements, videos, and briefs to educate the public about PHC and invite their support and participation in effecting changes in the acute-care oriented health care system. Projects in Newfoundland and Quebec have involved the public directly in providing health promotion and illness prevention activities within their communities (Rodger & Gallagher, 1995). Public forums, position papers, and lobbying have been used extensively by all nursing associations to educate and involve the public.

The principles of PHC toward which the least efforts have been made by the nursing associations are intersectoral and interdisciplinary collaboration and appropriate technology. Although there have been concerted efforts to cooperate and collaborate with the traditional health professions and within the health care system, few activities reported have addressed intersectoral collaboration with organizations and groups outside the system. Two examples cited by Rodger and Gallagher (1995) are RNABC's involvement in bicycle helmet and safe drinking water projects and Newfoundland nurses' participation in a community substance abuse program and other projects with school personnel and the Royal Canadian Mounted Police. Rodger and Gallagher (1995) conclude that intersectoral collaboration is the area requiring the greatest effort by community health nurses and nursing at large. With the increasing use of technologies in the home as well as in hospitals, there is no doubt that nurses need to be involved in discussions of their use and appropriateness. Some organizations are addressing this principle through publications to educate members and for use in educating the public and in lobbying. The Saskatchewan Registered Nurses Association has a representative on the Health Minister's Technology Advisory Committee as one means of influencing the dissemination and use of technologies (Rodger & Gallagher, 1995).

■ Socioeconomic Determinants of Health

To attain the goal of Health for All, health care planners must consider the influence of socioeconomic determinants of health. The determinants include such factors as poverty, racism, violence, pollution, and stigmatization. All have deleterious effects on the health of individuals and families and on their ability to develop effective problem solving and coping skills. Such factors have a profound influence on the health care needs of communities.

Poverty is a major deterrent to health by placing individuals and families at greater risk of contracting diseases and disabling chronic conditions and of being exposed to environmental hazards, such as violence in the home and community and pollution in poor living conditions. Reutter (1995) reports that "in 1992, 16% of Canadians were living below the poverty line" (p. 224). Certain groups within the population are at greater risk of being poor. These include women heads of single parent families, 58% of whom had incomes below the poverty line in 1992. In some cases the women have left an abusive relationship after years of abuse and have limited job skills as well as being unable to afford child care. Persons at both ends of the life span are also at greater risk of being poor with 18% of children being impoverished in 1992 and 43% of all poor children living in single-parent families headed by a mother (National Council of Welfare, 1994). Another vulnerable group within the Canadian population is unattached senior women who are represented disproportionately within the 19% of all seniors living below the poverty line. The results of discrimination against women in the job market and in salary levels are clearly reflected in these data. Even though the Canadian health care system is supposed to be universally accessible to all citizens, Badgley (1991) reports that this is not always the case. For example, a study of homeless adults in Toronto revealed that even though almost 40% had Ontario health insurance, 7% had been refused care; some reported that their problems were not investigated fully and that they were treated rudely; and 25% were unable to carry out instructions in their deprived living conditions (Crowe, 1993).

Poverty is known to be related to birth outcomes with infants from poor neighbourhoods being 30% to 50% more likely to be premature, of low birth weight, or retarded in development than infants born into richer homes (Wilkins, Sherman & Best, 1989). They were also much more likely to die during the postneonatal period or during the first year of life. Studies have also shown that poor children are at greater risk of dying from accidents, poisoning, and violence (Avard & Hanvey, 1989; Dougherty, Pless, & Wilkins, 1990; Wilkins, Adams, & Brancker, 1989). Children from poor families are also more likely to have chronic health problems, mental and physical disabilities, and to be at greater risk of poor school performance and less likely to continue on to postsecondary school education (Ryerse, 1990). Poor school performance may be related to inadequate nutrition as well as to lack of support and supervision in the home. Poor children are also at greater risk of abuse and neglect although child abuse and wife abuse happen in families of all social strata.

Reutter (1995) identifies racial and ethnic minorities as high risk populations, particularly the Aboriginal population whose incomes were reported to be approximately ⅔ of non-Aboriginal averages. Shah (1990) found that only about half the adult Aboriginal population was in the labour force and predominantly in low-paying service industries. In addition, there may be biases toward cultural minorities that influence adversely their access to services and the quality of care delivered. Caregivers' lack of knowledge of cultural beliefs and practices may serve as further deterrents to the provision of quality health care services.

Other barriers to accessibility to care are geographic location, which results in social isolation, and stigmatized populations with health problems, such as HIV/AIDS, who may encounter biases that influence the quality of care adversely. Such vulnerable individuals and groups are not only at greater risk but also may feel disenfranchised and lack the social supports necessary to effectively manage an emotionally and physically healthy lifestyle (Sebastian, 1992). Sebastian (1992) points out that "vulnerable groups have limited involvement in the health planning to meet their own needs. Because these groups are primarily minorities, they are more disadvantaged than most mainstream groups because typical health planning focuses on the majority" (pp. 3-4).

Vulnerable groups lack control over financial resources, which limits their choices among available options within the health care system. They also may lack knowledge of health care resources and access to social networks, both of which would help them to use health care resources more effectively. Although not all vulnerable groups or individuals have limited education, many have. This serves as another deterrent to their attaining and maintaining healthy lifestyles. This multiplicity of factors combined with lack of political skills, places vulnerable individuals and groups at a disadvantage in relation to influencing change in health care systems.

■ Change in the Canadian Health Care System

For almost a decade all provinces have been examining models of health care to better incorporate principles of PHC and better meet the needs of their constituencies, as well as address financial problems. This has been done through advisory committees, task forces, or commissions who invited input from the public and health care groups. Organized nursing has taken advantage of the opportunities and their input is reflected in the provincial reports. Mhatre and Deber (1992) critically analysed the policy options set forth in the reports and identified a number of recurring themes, some of which reflect the principles of PHC and the directions proposed by nursing to better meet the health care needs of citizens and better utilize nursing resources. Following are the recurring themes:

1. Broadening the definition of health with the collaboration of multiple sectors.
2. Shifting emphasis from curing illness to promoting health and preventing disease.
3. Switching focus to community-based rather than institution-based care.
4. Providing more opportunity for individuals to participate with service providers in making decisions on health choices and policies.
5. Devolution or decentralization of the provincial systems to some form of regional authorities.
6. Improved human resources planning, with particular emphasis on alternative methods for remuneration of physicians.
7. Enhanced efficiency in the management of services through the establishment of councils, coordinating bodies, and secretariats.

8. Increasing funds for health services research, especially in the areas of utilization, technology assessment, program/system evaluation, and information systems (Mhatre & Deber, 1992, p. 655).

These themes were identified in the reports resulting from extensive reviews of the health care systems in 6 of the 10 Canadian provinces (Alberta, New Brunswick, Nova Scotia, Ontario, Quebec, and Saskatchewan). Although all of the themes were not mentioned in all of the reports, it is encouraging to note that all 6 provinces identified the need for a broader definition of health; shifting emphasis to health promotion and disease prevention; changing emphasis to community-based care; increasing participation of nonproviders of care in decision making; developing regional authorities to facilitate achievement of consumer participation, community-based care, equity of services, and improved efficiency and effectiveness; and improved human resources planning. All provinces, except Alberta, identified the need to examine alternative methods for remunerating physicians, a change not likely to be supported by physicians. Changes are already occurring in some provinces, such as Alberta, where regional authorities are already being organized. It is important for nursing organizations and nurses as individuals to continue to monitor and be involved in the planning and effecting of changes to ensure that the principles of PHC are upheld as well as the 5 principles of the Canada Health Act.

■ Opportunities for Nursing Leadership in Primary Health Care

Nursing leaders in all national and provincial/territorial nursing organizations have demonstrated strong commitment to promoting and facilitating attainment of the goals of PHC. It is important that all nurses support them in working toward that goal and in lobbying to influence change in health policy in Canada. There is increasing evidence of support to make more nurses a point of entry to the health-care system and reallocate health-care funds to support primary health care. Changes will be required in both the health care system and nursing education, to enable nurses to provide leadership and function more effectively.

To achieve this goal, nurses must be prepared to accept shared responsibility with people for their own health, rather than use the traditional, authoritative approach as providers of care. Nurses must be willing to support communities in addressing matters concerning their health, lifestyles, and well-being. They must develop new skills in empowering people for self-care, self-help, and environmental improvement and in promoting healthy coping strategies to maintain health (Maglacas, 1988).

Nursing educators must examine curricula to ensure that they are teaching the concept of PHC as previously interpreted. This is particularly important if the findings of two studies of nursing education programs are representative of all programs in Canada. The purposes of a study by Edwards and Craig (1987) were to determine

(1) the primary health-care concepts in Canadian nursing curricula; (2) faculty's familiarity with primary health-care concepts; (3) the perceived importance of a primary health-care focus in various settings; and (4) the extent to which primary health-care concepts are taught by nursing educators. Their findings revealed that 31.4% of the respondents were aware of the Alma-Ata Declaration, and 19.6% had read the ICN statement on PHC. Approximately 88% were unaware of the Canadian government position on PHC. Responses indicated poor differentiation between the concepts of primary care, primary nursing, and PHC. The inclusion of PHC knowledge and skills was minimal and significantly less than expected.

Tenn and Niskala (1992) conducted a survey of Canadian university faculties/schools of nursing to determine the extent and nature of incorporation of PHC in curricula. Responses were received from 31 of the 32 organizations eligible to participate. The findings revealed that about 60% of the faculties/schools have integrated primary health care in their curricula to a reasonable degree and that "some have been highly successful in their integration, especially those who designed their curricula with primary health care as the basis" (p. 49). Most programs integrate the principle of health promotion and disease prevention in relation to individuals, families, and groups and support a partnership role for the nurse working with individuals and families; however, the principle of public participation and empowerment as a strategy to facilitate participation, were rarely included. Further, the clinical experiences available are not usually conducive to promoting public participation. They found that the principle of intersectoral collaboration "seemed to be integrated to a reasonable degree in most programs" but did not comment on the availability of clinical experiences to implement this principle. Finding appropriate practice opportunities in PHC seemed to present a problem for many faculties/schools who placed students in traditional settings (hospitals, health units, and long-term care facilities), rather than seeking out new settings such as group homes, citizen groups, youth organizations, coalitions for community action, and PHC projects. The findings of this study identify some needs for change in curricula to better prepare nursing students to learn and apply the principles of PHC in practice.

■ The Future of Primary Health Care

The opportunities for nurses to practise PHC, as envisioned by CNA, the provincial/territorial nursing associations, Maglacas, and other nursing leaders, are unlimited if they believe in the concept and accept the challenge to work with communities in promoting and facilitating implementation of the principles of PHC. As we move forward into the 21st century, if ever there was a need for unity in nursing, this is the time to advance the cause of PHC. To attain nursing's goals and achieve Health for All by the year 2000, will require major changes in the health-care system and reorientation of perceptions of nursing and the education needed to function effectively in the future. As nurses, why not join forces with the public and work toward these goals?

■ REFERENCES

Alberta Association of Registered Nurses. (1993). *Nurses: Key to healthy Albertans: Position of AARN on increased direct access to services provided by registered nurses* (ed 2). Edmonton: The Association.

Alberta Association of Registered Nurses. (1993). *Nurses: Key to healthy Albertans: A proposal for change.* Brochure available from 11620 - 168 St., Edmonton, Alberta T5M 4A6.

Alberta Association of Registered Nurses. (1993). *Nurses: Key to healthy Albertans.* Booklet available from 11620-168 St., Edmonton, Alberta T5M A46.

Alberta Association of Registered Nurses. (1994). Update of AARN initiative on increased direct access to services provided by registered nurses. *AARN Newsletter, 50*(2), 12-13.

Allen, M. (1977). Comparative theories of the expanded role and implications for nursing practice. *Nursing Papers, 9*(2), 38-45.

Allen, M. (1981). The health dimension in nursing practice: Notes on nursing and primary health care. *Journal of Advanced Nursing, 6*(3), 63-64.

Allen, M. (1983). Primary care nursing: Research in action. In L. Hockey (Ed.), *Primary care nursing* (pp. 32-77). Edinburgh: Churchill Livingstone.

Association of Registered Nurses of Newfoundland. (1987). *Primary health care: A nursing model: An overview.* St. John's, Newfoundland: The Association.

Avard, D., & Hanvey, L. (1989). *The health of Canada's children: A CICH profile.* Ottawa: Canadian Institute of Child Health.

Badgley, R. F. (1991). Social and economic disparities under Canadian health care. *International Journal of Health Services, 21*(4), 659-671.

Canadian Nurses Association. (1988). *Health for all Canadians: A call for health care reform.* Ottawa: The Association.

Canadian Nurses Association. (1989). *Position statement on the nurse's role in primary health care.* Ottawa: The Association.

Canadian Nurses Association. (1995). *Policy statement on the role of the nurse in primary health care.* Ottawa: The Association.

Chamberlain, M. C., & Beckingham, A. C. (1987). Primary health care in Canada: In praise of the nurse? *International Nursing Review, 34*(6), 158-160.

Chambers, L. W., & West, A. E. (1978). The St. John's randomized trial of the family practice nurse: Health outcomes of patients. *International Journal of Epidemiology, 7*(2), 153-161.

CNA Connection. (1988). Keynote speaker: Empowerment key role says Maglacas. *The Canadian Nurse, 84*(8), 14-15.

CNA Connection. (1989). CNA board endorses primary health care. *The Canadian Nurse, 85*(5), 8.

Crowe, C. (1993). Nursing research and political change: The Street health report. *The Canadian Nurse, 89*(1), 21-24.

Denton, F., Gafini, D., Spencer, B., & Stoddart, G. (1982). *Potential savings from the adoption of nurse practitioner technology in the Canadian health care system.* Hamilton, Ontario: McMaster University.

Diers, D., Hamman, A., & Molde, S. (1986). Complexity of ambulatory care: Nurse practitioner and physician caseloads. *Nursing Research, 35*(5), 310-314.

Dougherty, G., Pless, B., & Wilkins, R. (1990). Social class and the occurrence of traffic injuries and deaths in urban children. *Canadian Journal of Public Health, 81,* 204-209.

Edwards, N. C., & Craig, H. (1987). *Does nursing education reflect the goals of primary health care?* Hamilton, Ontario: McMaster University.

Feldman, M. J., Ventura, M. R., & Crosby, F. (1987). Studies of nurse practitioner effectiveness. *Nursing Research, 36*(5), 303-308.

Flett, J. E., Last, J. M., & Lynch G. U. (1980). Evaluation of the public health nurse as primary health care provider for elderly people. In V. Marshall (Ed.), *Aging in Canada: Social perspectives* (pp. 177-188). Don Mills, Ontario: Fitzhenry and Whiteside.

Innes, J. (1987). Health care reform: Sketching the future. *AARN Newsletter, 43*(8), 1, 5-6.

Jamieson, M. K. (1990). Block nursing: Practicing autonomous professional nursing in the community. *Nursing & Health Care, 11,* 250-253.

Kassakian, M. G., Bailey, L. R., Rinker, M., Stewart, C. A., & Yates, J. W. (1979). Cost and quality of dying: A comparison of home and hospital. *Nurse Practitioner, 4*(2), 18-23.

Maglacas, A. M. (1988). Health for all: Nursing's role. *Nursing Outlook, 36*(2), 66-71.

Mahler, H. (1981). The meaning of health for all by the year 2000. *World Health Forum, 2*(1), 5-22.

Mhatre, S. L., & Deber, R. B. (1992). From equal access to health care to equitable access to health: A review of Canadian provincial health commissions and reports. *International Journal of Health Services, 22*(4), 645-668.

Molde, S., & Diers, D. (1985). Nurse practitioner review: Selected literature review and research agenda. *Nursing Research, 34*(6), 362-367.

National Council of Welfare. (1994). *Poverty profile: 1992.* Ottawa: Minister of Supply and Services Canada.

Nutbeam, D., & Lawrence, J. (1987). *Positive health: An update on health promotion in action: A charter for action.* Cardiff: Institute for Health Promotion, College of Medicine, University of Wales.

Ottawa Charter for Health Promotion. (1986). Ottawa: World Health Organization, Health and Welfare Canada, and the Canadian Public Health Association.

Ramsay, J., McKenzie, J. K., & Fish, D. G. (1982). Physicians and nurse practitioners: Do they provide equivalent care? *American Journal of Public Health, 72*(4), 55-57.

Report of the Committee on Nurse Practitioners. (1972). Ottawa: Department of National Health and Welfare, The Committee.

Reutter, L. I. (1995). Socioeconomic determinants of health. In M.J. Stewart (Ed.), *Community nursing: Promoting Canadians' health* (pp. 223-245). Toronto: W.B. Saunders.

Rodger, G. L. & Gallagher, S. M. (1995). The move toward primary health care in Canada: Community health nursing from 1985 to 1995. In M.J. Stewart (Ed.), *Community nursing: Promoting Canadians' health* (pp. 37-58). Toronto: WB Saunders.

Ryerse, C. (1990). *Thursday's child: Child poverty in Canada: A review of the effects of poverty on children.* Ottawa: National Youth in Care Network.

Sadoway, D. T., Plan, R. H. M., & Soskolne, C. L. (1990). Infant and preschool immunization delivery in Alberta and Ontario: A partial cost-minimization analysis. *Canadian Journal of Public Health, 81*(2), 146-151.

Sebastian, J. G. (1992). Vulnerable populations in the community: In M. Stanhope & J. Lancaster (Eds.), *Community health nursing: Process and practice for promoting health* (pp. 365-390). St. Louis: Mosby-Year Book.

Spitzer, W., Kergin, D. J., & Yoshida, M. A. (1975). Nurse practitioners in primary care: The southern Ontario randomized trial. In M. Leininger (Ed.), *Health care dimensions.* Philadelphia: F.A. Davis Company.

Shah, C. (1990). *Public health and preventive medicine in Canada* (ed 2). Toronto: University of Toronto Press.

Tenn, L., & Niskala, H. (1994). *Primary health care in the curricula of Canadian university schools of nursing.* (Final report to the Canadian Nurses' Foundation). Vancouver: University of British Columbia School of Nursing.

Thibaudeau, M. F., & Reidy, M. M. (1977). Nursing makes a difference: A comparative study of the health behaviours of mothers in three primary care agencies. *International Journal of Nursing Studies, 14,* 97-107.

Ulin, P. R. (1982). International nursing challenge. *Nursing Outlook, 30*(6), 531-535.

Warner, M. (1981). The health workshop: A nursing model of primary health care in a rural community. *The Canadian Nurse, 77*(1), 34-36.

Wilkins, R., Adams, O., & Brancker, A. (1989). Changes in mortality by income in urban Canada from 1971 to 1986. *Health Reports, 1*(2), 173-174.

Wilkins, R., Sherman, G., & Best, P. (1991). Birth outcomes and infant mortality by income in urban Canada, 1986. *Health Reports, 3*(1), 7-31.

World Health Organization. (1978a). *Report of the international conference on primary health care.* Alma-Ata, USSR, Geneva, September 6-12, 1978.

World Health Organization. (1978b). The Alma-Ata conference on primary health care. *WHO Chronicle, 32*(11), 409-430.

4 Primary Health Care and the Health of Families

Linda Reutter and Margaret J. Harrison

Primary health care (PHC) is identified by the World Health Organization as the means for achieving an acceptable standard of health for people worldwide using current resources. Following discussion on inequities in health care at the Thirtieth World Health Assembly in 1977, the World Health Organization met at Alma-Ata in an international conference on PHC. The Alma-Ata conference published the following definition of PHC: "essential health care made universally accessible to individuals and families, through their full participation, and at a cost the community and the country can afford" (WHO, 1978). The principles of PHC as the basis of health planning were reaffirmed by the World Health Organization at Riga in 1988 (WHO, 1988). With increasing concern about the cost of the present Canadian health-care system, there has been discussion among governments, health professionals, health economists, and the public about reforming the health-care system. The Canadian Nurses Association (CNA) has taken a stand in support of PHC as the means to achieve "Health for All." To outline its position, CNA has prepared several documents (CNA, 1988; CNA, 1989) in which they propose that nurses be active participants in a health-care system organized on PHC principles.

The five principles of PHC are accessibility of services, increased emphasis on prevention and promotion, lay participation, intersectoral cooperation, and appropriate technology. The principle of accessibility refers to the availability of essential care to the whole community in a manner that is acceptable to them. Using this principle, health care would be planned to address inequities in health care experienced by groups in the community. PHC focuses on health rather than illness. This goal is achieved by placing an emphasis on promotive and preventive care rather than curative care in the planning and provision of health services. In implementing the principle of lay participation, consumers become active partners with professionals, administrators, and governments in health-care planning, delivery, and evaluation. The principle of intersectoral cooperation highlights the contribution of non-health agencies to the health of a nation. Health is linked closely to the economic, educational, and physical environments in which people live and work. Therefore health care is best achieved when the social and economic sectors of the community work cooperatively with the health-care sector. To provide accessible services equitably to the community, primary health-care principles promote the use of technology that is affordable to the community and available to all.

Although some Canadian nurses have provided PHC in the past, there has been an increasing focus on PHC in recent years. This chapter describes recent trends in nursing in Canada which reflect the principles of PHC. The recognition of the importance of PHC principles in planning health programs raises a number of issues for nursing practice. This chapter also discusses issues in nursing education related to the increasing emphasis on PHC.

■ Current Examples of Primary Health Care in Canada

PHC principles are evident in many nursing activities in Canada (see CNA, 1988; 1992 for examples). Some of the PHC activities occur in traditional settings, while other PHC projects are located in innovative and unique settings. Because PHC is not only an approach to providing health-care services but also a concept of health care (WHO, 1978; Krebs, 1983), the principles can be applied to some degree within existing structures and services.

Before discussing current examples of nurses working in PHC services, it should be noted that some Canadian nurses had been incorporating principles of PHC before the Alma-Ata conference. In particular, public health nurses provided care to individuals and families that was community based and had a preventive or health promotion focus. Members of the community were involved in planning and administering these programs. In addition, nurses working in northern and remote areas worked with small communities to provide health care with minimal resources. Other nurses emphasized the importance of self-care practices and contributions to her well being at an individual level. The following discussion of the role of nurses in PHC includes selected examples from settings in which PHC principles have traditionally been practised, as well as settings that are innovative.

Public Health Nursing Services

The work of public health nurses (PHNs) in public health units incorporates the principles of PHC (Jones & Craig, 1988; Mills & Ready, 1988). Public health science addresses human health within the broader context of the life process of the community. PHNs are concerned with providing comprehensive, essential services to the entire community, with an emphasis on health promotion and the prevention of illness and injury. While public health nursing's concern is the health of the total community, there is a strong emphasis on family health promotion. Client self-determination is a key concept in public health nursing.

Increasingly, the social determinants of health are seen as legitimate targets of nursing interventions, as PHNs work collaboratively with other disciplines and non-health sectors to promote healthy public policy. Collaboration occurs through organizations such as the Canadian Public Health Association (CPHA). This interdisciplinary organization, in its Position Paper on Healthy Public Policy (CPHA 1989), recognized that Canadians varied in their opportunities to have access to food, shelter, work, education, and income. CPHA argues that these inequities could be addressed through changes in public policy (CPHA, 1990). PHNs through provincial branches of the Community Health Nurses Association of Canada have also become more active in determining healthy public policy by presenting to government organizations the roles that they fulfill in the community and the issues that are faced by families with whom they work.

PHNs are involved in working with community groups to identify and meet community needs at the community level. However, they have identified that PHNs need better preparation in community development skills to function effectively in this role (Working Group, 1991).

To make health care "culturally accessible" to aboriginal peoples, PHNs may be assisted by community health representatives. For example, in Whitehorse, Yukon, the local First Nations Community has its own health clinic, staffed by one nurse and community health representatives, who are employed by and accountable to the band. The programs at the clinic are directed toward the needs of this particular community (CNA, 1992).

Centres with Outreach to Underserved Populations

Two agencies that use a multidisciplinary team to make health care more accessible to the inner city population are the Centretown Community Health Centre in Ottawa and the Boyle-McCauley Health Centre in Edmonton, Alberta. In both centres, physicians are in salaried positions and the centre is governed by a board of community representatives.

During the 1980s the Centretown Community Health Centre board and staff recognized a shift in the population that they served with increasing numbers of impoverished individuals living in rooming houses and on the street. The Centre has developed an outreach program in which nurses make weekly visits to two community drop-in centres. The services provided by the nurses include health assessments, health education, and referrals to other agencies. Nurses working in this program also work with other organizations to address issues such as poor housing, illiteracy, and unemployment (personal communication, Jane McDonald, August 1993).

Boyle-McCauley Health Centre (BMHC) is a street-front, walk-in clinic whose main mission is to provide easily accessible health care to an inner-city community. This agency also demonstrates many principles of PHC. Its services include both medical care and health care directed toward health promotion and illness and injury prevention. The BMHC employs nurse practitioners, physicians, dietitians, volunteers, mental health consultants, psychologists, and addictions counselors. Staff at the BMHC collaborate closely with other inner-city agencies. The services provided are based on the needs of the community and include such programs as needle exchanges, a foot care clinic, and mental health counseling. In addition to providing clinic services, home visits are conducted by three nurses to provide primary care, health assessment, and health education to seniors, expectant and new mothers, and chronically ill individuals. In a similar manner as the Centretown Community Health Centre, staff at BMHC attempt to contact others who need health care through outreach programs in rooming houses and half-way houses. BMHC is presently in the process of securing funding for a dental clinic. The involvement of BMHC in a community economic development project exemplifies the agency's understanding of and commitment to the interrelationship between health and social and economic development (BMHC, 1993).

Victorian Order of Nurses

The Victorian Order of Nurses (VON) is a voluntary agency with a PHC philosophy and a long history of innovation in meeting the needs of the community. VON provides community services that promote, maintain, and improve health and enhance independence and quality of life. A recently completed project called PEP (Promoting Elders Participation) involved seniors in rural underserved areas in assessing their needs and establishing services to meet them. Another VON initiative is the VON primary health-care clinic in Lark Harbour, Newfoundland. This clinic was built by local residents and meets community needs such as seniors' health counseling, fitness, weight control, foot care clinics, and prenatal education and follow-up (VON, 1992b). The VON is also part of a new "Quick Response Program" in two Windsor, Ontario hospitals. Collaboration with other agencies, such as hospitals, home care programs, and visiting homemaker agencies, helps prevent hospital admissions. When seniors arrive in emergency departments, they are assessed and if possible sent home where a team of health-care workers can be mobilized to prevent institutionalization (VON, 1992a).

Nurses as Access to Health Care

A new health-care program that expands the scope of nursing practice in the area of PHC is the McAdam Project in New Brunswick, opened in 1993. This project provides both community health-care programs and emergency services under one roof. Nurses coordinate the service, complete the initial client history, assess and analyze health-care needs, provide care, and refer clients to other professionals as needed. The physician involved in the project is part of the team and has a salaried position. Community health services are currently being developed based on a community needs assessment by a nurse. Future services may include well-child clinics, developmental screening, and immunization clinics. Nurses will also be involved in providing outreach services and developing links with existing community resources. A multidisciplinary team, including members of the community, will continue to evaluate community needs and develop further programs with available resources (Penny Short, personal communication, August 1993).

The Registered Nurses Association of Nova Scotia is cosponsoring with the Department of Health and the Sacred Heart Hospital a three year primary health-care project in Cheticamp, Nova Scotia. In this project, which commenced in November 1992, the nurse is the primary health-care provider and gives direct care in addition to providing health education to health personnel and the public, acting as an advocate for the community and managing and supervising the primary health-care services (Parent, 1993).

■ Issues in PHC

This overview of current services in Canada that incorporate PHC principles suggests that nurses are well positioned to incorporate PHC principles into their nursing practice. Before nurses are able to fully participate in health-care delivery, however, there is a need to establish an overall strategy for health in Canada, with clear objectives and goals (CPHA, 1992; RNABC, 1990a). Until a national plan for health care is developed, the following issues remain which prevent or threaten the full realization of PHC.

Removing Financial Barriers to Accessible Health Care

In spite of Canada's universal health-care insurance, many essential health services are not publicly insured, thus making accessibility income-dependent. For example, working low-income families may not receive extended health-care benefits from their employers, including dental care, prescription drugs, special medical needs, and optometry. Premiums for these services, in addition to the regular health premiums, may be too costly for families who are already at or near the poverty line (FSA and ISAC, 1992). Cutbacks in Aids to Living equipment may minimize the self-care and reliance of physically disabled individuals in the community (RNABC, 1990a). At a time when "stress" is the major health concern for many Canadians (Health and Welfare Canada, 1993), it is noteworthy that mental health counseling services by other than physicians are not insured to the same extent as services provided by psychiatrists in provinces such as Alberta.

Although the impetus for restructuring the health-care system toward a PHC model comes in part from the rising costs of health care, the current fiscal crisis precipitated by an increasingly burdensome public debt may undermine important PHC concepts that are currently protected by the Canada Health Act. For example, the introduction of user fees in Canada currently being discussed to offset rising health-care costs may create financial barriers to accessible health care, particularly for those on fixed incomes. Privatization of health-care services may also contribute to a "two-tiered" health-care system. The CNA has argued that there is a need for nurses to become politically active in preserving a Canadian health-care system that is universally accessible, comprehensive, portable, and publicly administered (CNA, August 1993).

Determining Essential Services

Essential health care includes a range of services encompassing promotion, prevention, rehabilitation, and support, in addition to curative services (WHO, 1978). Each of these areas should receive the level of resources that reflects its contributions to the health of the population (CNA, 1988; RNABC, 1990a). When resources are limited, only curative services may be considered essential, with the result that needed rehabilitation and health promotion services are underfunded. With the introduction of short-stay hospital programs, more acutely ill clients are being discharged into the community. While this is an important step in providing health care closer to home, adequate community resources must be in place to support these individuals. Without increased funding at the community level to accommodate this shift, existing resources in the community may be reallocated to care for the immediate needs of these clients to the potential neglect of health promotion and illness prevention services.

Although many federal and provincial government health documents incorporate PHC principles (Epp, 1986; Premier's Commission, 1989), inadequate resources are often allocated to community-based care, particularly health promotion and disease prevention. In Canada, only 3% to 5% of health expenditures are allocated to health promotion and community health services (CNA, 1988). RNABC (1990b) in its submission to the Royal Commission of Health Care and Costs pointed out that the core programs provided by public health units to support family health, while directed to primary prevention and health promotion of all families, are increasingly being directed only toward high-risk families because of inadequate funding.

Appropriate Use of Personnel

Socially acceptable and affordable methods of health-care delivery include administrative and organizational structures such as method of payment of health-care professionals and the appropriate use of personnel. Nurses have argued that health care in Canada could be made more accessible and affordable through expansion of the nurse's role in providing health services and by providing clients with direct access to nursing services (RNABC, 1990a; CNA, 1988, 1993; AARN, 1993). Nurses, as a point of entry to the health-care system, are prepared to do initial assessments, help clients define needs, work with clients in meeting these needs, and direct clients to the most appropriate care providers. In its emphasis on health-care reform, the CNA is concentrating on the unique role that nurses can play in making quality health care accessible and affordable without compromising the five principles of Canada's medicare system. This expanded role is rooted in health promotion and illness prevention and therefore is much more than the assumption of selected medical functions of physicians.

Vested interests of professionals in their traditional roles, however, may make it difficult for nurses to expand their roles, and for these nursing services to become publicly insurable and directly accessible to clients. For example, the practice of midwifery in British Columbia (RNABC, 1990a) and Alberta until 1992 was blocked by the medical practitioners. Recognition must also be given to the role of nonprofessionals and traditional practitioners in providing entry to the health-care system. Nurses need to support the use of community health workers and traditional practitioners to make care more culturally accessible and relevant (Shestowsky, 1992).

An interesting issue in relation to the appropriate use of personnel has arisen in the McAdam project previously discussed. Here the Minister of Health, physicians, and nurses agree on the expanded scope of nursing practice with nurses as direct access to the health-care system. However, such involvement would require changes to the Hospital Services Act. In this situation, professionals are constrained by existing legislation and a reticence to open the Act (Penny Short, personal communication).

Broadening the Concept of Health

In addition to providing access to health care, PHC emphasizes the importance of the relationship between health and the economic and social dimensions of a community. Health is concerned with overall human development and is viewed as a resource that enables people to live socially and economically productive lives (WHO, 1984). Many major health problems faced by families in Canada today, such as family violence and substance abuse, are embedded in social environments. The adverse effects of poverty on individual, family, and community health are well documented (Blackburn, 1991; Kaplan-Sanoff et al., 1991; Wilkins, 1988). Political, social, and cultural forces operate to affect health status directly by limiting access to conditions conducive to health, as well as through their influence on personal health behaviours. It is important for nurses to recognize that individual choices are influenced by environmental supports and constraints. To change environments to become health-enhancing rather than health-inhibiting, nurses may need to use social action strategies that target social institutions rather than individuals. A socioecological view of health also acknowledges that policies in non-health sectors influence community health; therefore, intersectoral collaboration is required to ensure that all public policy enhances health.

Nurses have traditionally used individualistic models of health behaviour and change to enhance individual and family health (Butterfield, 1990). Such approaches use psychological theories to explain patterns of health and health care (Dreher, 1982) and focus on altering client attitudes and knowledge rather than altering the environment or empowering clients to do so (Butterfield, 1990). An "upstream" focus to preventing family health problems will require thinking more broadly about the economic, political, and environmental factors that inhibit health. New approaches and theoretical frameworks that consider the social determinants of health, such as critical social theory, could provide direction for nursing interventions at a societal level (Stevens & Hall, 1992; Kleffel, 1991; Kristjanson & Chalmers, 1991).

Developing Collaboration

All of the major documents on PHC discuss the need for collaborative work. Collaboration includes collaboration between clients (mutual aid), clients and practitioners (self-determination), practitioners (integrated service), practitioners and communities (community development), and communities and governments (building healthy public policy) (RNABC, 1990a). The PHC principle that clients are active participants in identifying and meeting their health needs may require a shift in nurses' perceptions of the nurse-client interaction. For collaboration to work, health-care practitioners must be willing to trust people and communities to be responsible for their own health and to "do with" rather than "do to." Becoming a partner in care rather than a provider of care will require consulting, enabling, and facilitating skills. Current nursing frameworks, such as those developed by Orem (1985) and Neuman (1989), will assist in this change when working with individuals, as these frameworks emphasize client autonomy and self-determination. Working collaboratively with families in a partner relationship is emphasized in the community health nursing literature (e.g., Kristjanson & Chalmers, 1991; Pesznecker, Zerwekh, & Horn, 1989).

Perhaps a greater gap in the area of collaboration between nurses and clients is in relation to informal support networks (Stewart, 1990). A study of the learning needs of a sector of Canadian nurses regarding lay support groups reported that nurses had inadequate knowledge of specific mutual aid groups and the benefits and characteristics of self-help and community organization and consulting skills (Stewart, 1989). Collaboration also involves collaborating with other health disciplines. This may be difficult if disciplines including nursing maintain vested interests and proceed from an adversarial position. For PHC to work, there must be free and open lines of referral among health and social service providers.

■ Implications for Nursing Education

For nursing educators there are implications in the current movement towards a more active role for nurses in delivering primary health care (Innes, 1987). The findings of an early study by Edwards and Craig (1987) indicated that the inclusion of PHC knowledge and skills in Canadian nursing curricula was minimal and significantly less than expected. Only 31.4% of nursing educators were aware of the Alma-Ata declaration and 19.6% had read the ICN statement on primary health care; 88% were unaware of the Canadian government's position on PHC. Moreover, responses indicated poor differentiation between the concepts of primary care, primary nursing, and PHC.

A recent study was conducted by Tenn and Niskala (1994) to determine the extent to which Canadian university schools of nursing currently include PHC concepts in their undergraduate and graduate curricula. Approximately 60% of the schools were described as having a reasonable degree of integration of PHC in their curricula. Most programs include a health promotion focus and stress intersectoral collaboration for the health of individuals, families, and groups. Collaborative partnership roles with communities were less frequently included. Students rarely obtained clinical experience in settings conducive to public participation.

The definition of health and the importance of collaboration in PHC have implications for nursing education and for nursing practice models. The broad definition of health espoused by PHC means that students will require a solid foundation in epidemiology (particularly social epidemiology) and environmental health. Chalmers and Kristjanson (1989) suggest that the elective courses for nursing students have traditionally been from disciplines that maintain a predominant focus on the individual such as psychology. Elective course offerings that place greater emphasis on the social context of health and health behaviours, such as sociology or anthropology, need to be incorporated into curricula. In addition, to enhance healthy environments by meaningful interventions directed toward social structures, students will also require a sound knowledge of political systems and processes. Tenn and Niskala (1994) found Canadian schools of nursing had limited emphasis in their curricula on the partnership role of the nurse in acting on determinants of health.

Students will need to develop skills to collaborate with lay individuals and groups as well as with a variety of health and non-health professionals. The importance of collaboration with lay helpers is reflected in a conceptual framework for nursing education developed by Stewart (1990). Stewart found that most educational programs do not adequately develop the professional's skill in working with mutual aid and self-help groups. She advocates integrating social support theory into educational curricula to help professionals in their facilitative role with lay support groups.

It has been suggested that to facilitate harmonious working relationships among health professionals in intersectoral and interdisciplinary teams, opportunity should be provided for students to take interdisciplinary courses in their undergraduate programs (CNA, 1988). Interdisciplinary educational preparation of health professionals, however, is not widespread in Canada despite the success of pilot projects at McMaster, Manitoba, and other universities (CNA, 1988). Nurses continue to be educated for a single discipline mode.

To address some of these issues in their new undergraduate program, the University of Alberta Faculty of Nursing established an ad hoc committee on PHC and health promotion. This committee had representatives from the University of Alberta and the five collaborating diploma programs. The purpose of the committee was to ensure that PHC concepts are integrated throughout the 4-year program. Committee members monitored the curriculum implementation and acted as a resource for faculty members on PHC and health promotion principles. In addition, two interdisciplinary courses were developed, one in international health and the other in ethics in health care.

The McGill Model of Nursing

To assist students in applying PHC principles in their practice, a nursing framework that incorporates the principles of PHC should be selected. Moira Allen and her colleagues at McGill University have developed a Canadian nursing model that is consistent with some of the principles of PHC (Allen, 1983; Gottlieb & Rowat, 1987). This model has been called the Allen Nursing Model (Kravitz & Frey, 1989) or the McGill Model (Gottlieb & Rowat, 1987).

Moira Allen (1983) argued that the most effective use of nursing skill was not in a replacement role for physicians in the provision of illness care but rather in a complementary role in which nurses focused on the health of families and individuals. Allen believed that the role of nursing was in the promotion and facilitation of family health. The family was seen as the arena in which the individual learned how to maintain a healthy lifestyle. Unhealthy lifestyles had been identified as the cause of much of the illness and disability in Canada (Lalonde, 1974).

Nurses who use this model in their practice will provide care that reflects some of the principles of PHC. The primary goal of the McGill model is health promotion. The role of the nurse is to help the individual or family to acquire healthy ways of living and to develop skills in problem solving and coping. Although the definition of health in the McGill model is not as broad as the concept of health in primary health care, the McGill model shares the same emphasis on health care that is preventative or promotive rather than curative only.

In the McGill model, the family is seen as actively involved in seeking better health for its members and achieving life goals. The role of the nurse is that of a collaborator with the family. Rather than choosing or designing care for the family and the individual, the nurse works together with the family to choose goals and select approaches to care. Emphasis on the active participation of the public in collaboration with professionals in planning health services for communities is one of the principles of PHC. Nurses who work with families using the McGill model apply this principle at the individual and family level of care. As families are supported by nurses to become more skilled in problem solving, to develop improved coping skills and to live healthier lives, they also become more able to participate in community involvement in health-care planning. As this model addresses both health and illness using a health promotion focus, it has the potential to be used in acute care settings. The nurse and the family focus on health by assessing how the family is coping with the illness of an individual. Together they determine how the nurse could assist the family to develop further skill in problem solving and thus improve the family's coping.

The McGill model places less emphasis on the social and economic determinants of health than the concept of PHC. One of the principles of PHC is the integration of health with social and economic development. The environment in the McGill model refers to the settings in which learning can occur for the family: the home, the community, the workplace, and health-care agencies. The role of the nurse is to construct environments in which clients can learn to access information and resources. In this model the environment is the immediate circumstances or psychosocial environment of the family. Many of the health problems of families and the barriers to their ability to develop problem-solving skills and better coping lie in environmental conditions such as racism, poverty, violence, and pollution. In general, nursing models such as the McGill model have focused on an environmental paradigm that is client-oriented and psychosocial (Kleffel, 1991).

The McGill model evolved from descriptive studies of families in a variety of clinical settings. The goal of the model was to serve as a means of generating knowledge about nursing; Moira Allen expected the model to continue to develop over time based on research on the practice of nurses (Gottlieb & Rowat, 1987). Nurses may expand the McGill model of nursing in order to address environmental conditions that create barriers to the family's ability to learn new problem-solving skills and improved coping. As nurses increase their involvement in PHC, the concept of the environment in this model may change to include the role of the nurse in working in collaboration with families to identify and address the barriers in their environment which inhibit healthy living.

In summary, there is increasing emphasis on PHC as the means of providing universally accessible health care to Canadians. Nursing associations and nurses are developing a variety of services that provide nursing care using PHC principles. Despite the level of interest among nurses in providing PHC services, there remain a number of issues: the need to remove financial barriers for families to access health care, the need for health-care planners to define essential health-care services, the need to determine which health-care personnel are the appropriate source of care, the need to support a definition of health that includes economic and social conditions, and the need to develop collaboration between health disciplines and other sectors of the community. Nurses in practice and nursing educators have recognized the accompanying need for changes in the education of students and practitioners. Research on PHC principles in nursing education is currently being conducted and some educational programs have made changes to their curricula. With the continuing pressures on our health-care system, it is reasonable to expect further change in nursing practice and education.

■ REFERENCES

Alberta Association of Registered Nurses. (1993). *Nurses: Key to healthy Albertans.* Edmonton: The Association.
Allen, M. (1983). Primary care nursing: Research in action. In L. Hockey (Ed.). *Primary care nursing* (pp. 32-77). Edinburgh: Churchill Livingstone.
Blackburn, C. (1991). *Poverty and health: Working with families.* Milton Keynes: Open University Press.
Boyle-McCauley Health Centre (1993). *Annual update.* Edmonton: The Centre.
British Columbia Royal Commission on Health Care and Costs. (1991). *Closer to home.* Vancouver: Province of British Columbia.
Butterfield, P. (1990). Thinking upstream: Nurturing a conceptual understanding of the societal context of health behavior. *Advances in Nursing Science, 12*(2), 1-8.
Canadian Public Health Association. (1989). *Position paper on health public policy: A framework.* Ottawa: The Association.
Canadian Public Health Association. (1990). *Position paper on sustainability and equity: Primary health care in developing countries.* Ottawa: The Association.
Canadian Nurses Association. (1988). *Health care for all Canadians: A call for health-care reform.* Ottawa: The Association.
Canadian Nurses Association. (1989). *Position statement on primary health care.* Ottawa: The Association.
Canadian Nurses Association. (Nov./Dec. 1992). *CNA Today.* Ottawa: The Association.
Canadian Nurses Association. (May 1993). *CNA Today.* Ottawa: The Association.
Canadian Nurses Association. (August 1993). *CNA Today.* Ottawa: The Association.
Chalmers, K., & Kristjanson, L. (1989). The theoretical basis for nursing at the community level: A comparison of three models. *Journal of Advanced Nursing, 14,* 569-574.
Dreher, M. (1982). The conflict of conservatism in public health nursing education. *Nursing Outlook, 30,* 504-509.
Edwards, N. C., & Craig, H. (1987). *Does nursing education reflect the goals of primary health care?* Hamilton, ON: McMaster University.
Epp, J. (1986). *Achieving health for all: A health promotion framework.* Ottawa: Health and Welfare Canada.
Family Service Association of Edmonton and the Income Security Action Committee. (1991). *Working hard, living lean.* Edmonton: The Association.
Gottlieb, L. & Rowat, K. (1987). The McGill model of nursing: A practice-derived model. *Advances in Nursing Science, 9*(4), 51-61.
Innes, J. (1987). Health care reform: sketching the future. *AARN Newsletter, 43*(8), 1, 5-6.
Jones, P., & Craig, D. (1988). Nursing practice in the community: Primary health care. In A. Baumgart & J. Larsen (Eds.), *Canadian nursing faces the future* (pp. 135-149). Toronto: Mosby-Year Book.

Kaplan-Sanoff, M., Parker, S., & Zuckerman, B. (1991). Poverty and early childhood development: What do we know, and what should we do? *Infants and Young Children, 4*(1), 68-76.

Kleffel, D. (1991). Rethinking the environment as a domain of nursing knowledge. *Advances in Nursing Science, 14*(1), 40-51.

Kravitz, M. & Frey, M. A. (1989). The Allen Nursing Model. In J. Fitzpatrick & A. Whall (Eds.), *Conceptual models of nursing analysis and application* 2nd ed (pp. 313-329). East Norwalk, CT: Appleton & Lange.

Krebs, D. (1983). Nursing in primary health care. *International Nursing Review, 30*(5), 141-145.

Kristjanson, L. J. & Chalmers, K. (1991). Preventive work with families: Issues facing public health nurses. *Journal of Advanced Nursing, 16,* 147-153.

Lalonde M. (1974). *A new perspective on the health of Canadians.* Ottawa: Government of Canada.

Mills, K., & Ready, H. (1988). Health promotion in community nursing practice. In A. Baumgart & J. Larsen (Eds.), *Canadian nursing faces the future* (pp. 151-161). Toronto: Mosby-Year Book.

Neuman, B. (1989). *The Neuman systems model* ed. 2. Norfolk, CT: Appleton & Lange.

Orem, D. (1985). *Nursing: Concepts of practice* ed. 3. Toronto: McGraw-Hill.

Parent, K. (1993). The launch of the Cheticamp Primary Health Care Project. *Nurse to Nurse, 4*(1), 20-21.

Pesznecker, B., Zerwekh, R., & Horn, B. (1989). The mutual-participation relationship: Key to facilitating self-care practices in clients and families. *Public Health Nursing, 6,* 197-203.

Premier's Commission on Future Health Care for Albertans. (1989). *The Rainbow Report: Our vision for health.* Edmonton: The Association.

Registered Nurses Association of British Columbia. (1990a). *Primary health care: A discussion paper.* Vancouver: The Association.

Registered Nurses Association of British Columbia. (1990b). *Submission to the Royal Commission on Health Care and Costs.* Vancouver: The Association.

Shestowsky, B. (1992). *Traditional medicine and primary health care among Canadian aboriginal people.* Ottawa: Aboriginal Nurses Association of Canada.

Stephens, T. & Fowler, G. D. (Eds.). (1993). *Canada's Health Promotion Survey 1990: Technical report.* Ottawa: Health and Welfare Canada.

Stewart, M. J. (1989). Nurses' preparedness for health promotion through linkage with mutual-aid self-help groups. *Canadian Journal of Public Health, 80,* 110-114.

Stewart, M. J. (1990). From provider to provider: A conceptual framework for nursing education based on primary health care premises. *Advances in Nursing Science, 12*(2), 9-27.

Stevens, P., & Hall, J. (1992). Applying critical theories to nursing in communities. *Public Health Nursing, 9,* 2-9.

Tenn, L., & Niskala, H. (1994). *Primary health care in the curricula of Canadian university schools of nursing. Final report to the Canadian Nurses Foundation.* Vancouver, BC: University of British Columbia.

Victorian Order of Nurses (1992a). *Caring for life: Annual report 1991-92.* Ottawa: VON Canada.

Victorian Order of Nurses for Canada (1992b). *VON Canada Report.* Fall/Winter 1992. Ottawa: VON Canada.

Wilkins, R. (1988). *Special study on the socially and economically disadvantaged.* Ottawa: Minister of Supply and Services, Canada.

Working Group of Federal/Provincial/Territorial Nursing Consultants (1991). *Report of the working group on the educational requirements of community health nurses.* Ottawa: Health and Welfare.

World Health Organization (1978). *Primary health care: Report of the International Conference on Primary Health Care.* Alma-Ata, USSR, Geneva: WHO.

World Health Organization (1984). *Health promotion: A discussion document on the concept and principles.* Copenhagen: Regional Office for the World Health Organization.

World Health Organization (1988). *Alma-Ata reaffirmed at Riga.* Riga, USSR, Geneva: WHO.

5 ETHICAL AND LEGAL QUESTIONS IN NURSING PRACTICE

JANNETTA MACPHAIL AND JANET ROSS KERR

All citizens are responsible for their own actions under the law, and professionals have additional obligations to their clients by virtue of their specialized knowledge and skills. A professional whose performance of duties is believed by a client to be remiss may be called to account for actions in a court of law. In certain situations where an individual's actions are considered negligent, a suit may be brought by one person against another or in the case of a criminal matter, charges may be laid by the police. In our society it is commonly believed that people have certain ethical and moral obligations to one another. While some of these have been outlined in terms of general principles, obligations of an ethical or moral nature are generally less defined and clear-cut than those of a legal nature, as detailed descriptions of legal obligations between people under the law are spelled out in written form.

This is not the case with ethical relationships. Ethical dilemmas in health care are commonplace in an era in which lifesaving technology is widely available and in which awareness of ethical obligations between people is increasing. Indeed, people all over the world are increasingly coming to realize that people and nations, regardless of race, culture, and financial status cannot exist in isolation. All are dependent on others for survival ecologically. As pollution and other threatening life problems on the planet become more critical, relationships between nations will be mediated by the morality of relationships between people all over the world. In the perspective of the world as a global village, the economic environment may take a back seat to such developments.

Although legal and ethical issues in nursing are similar in Canada and the United States, the legal system and the application of ethical principles to nursing practice are unique in each country. Although the legal systems of both countries are based on English common law, differences in regulations, rules, and procedures governing the justice system, the courts, and professionals are considerable. In addition, although the traditions and trends of the law bear some similarity to one another, the cases from which precedents arise are clearly different in each country. Since ethics is much less clear-cut and involves difficult situations and dilemmas where it is difficult to reach readily acceptable solutions, in some ways developments in the United States and Canada have many common elements and developments are highly influential across borders. However, in presenting major ethical and legal issues in this chapter, the unique influence of the Canadian context forms the basis of the discussion.

Although health professionals have always encountered ethical issues and dilemmas in practise and have had to address difficult ethical questions, the issues and dilemmas today are highly complex. Factors contributing to this complexity are the rapidly expanding body of health care knowledge and the development of new technologies to save, generate, or prolong life. At the same time, changes in societal values have increased recognition of individual rights and freedoms and have heightened awareness of both the importance of and the need to protect those rights. Better-informed consumers who are more questioning and who expect to be more involved in decisions about their own lives and health have changed both the context and approaches to resolving ethical dilemmas. As a result of the eradication of many infectious and other diseases, improved control over still other diseases and improved living standards, human life span has been lengthened considerably over the course of this century. Because people are living longer, new ethical questions about the prolongation of life have been raised. Because health-care costs consume an increasing proportion of the Gross Domestic Product and because of the high cost of new technologies, society has realized that choices must be made in a climate of limited and finite resources. These questions about priorities in the health-care system and the best allocation of available resources require difficult decisions about who will receive care and under what conditions.

Health professionals face many dilemmas in everyday practice. Who decides what is right for the individual or family involved? Is there always a right answer? Curtin (1985, p. 1) defines ethics as "a discipline in which we attempt to identify, organize, analyze, and justify human acts by applying certain principles to determine the right thing to do in a given situation." Thus ethics is concerned with judgement of actions, not judgement of human beings. However, even when the best principles and the best intentions are applied to certain situations, the outcomes will not necessarily satisfy any or all of the parties involved. Because people are different, approaches and responses in similar but difficult ethical dilemmas are bound to be diverse.

■ Basic Ethical Theories and Principles

A prerequisite to applying ethics in nursing is having a theoretical base in ethics, just as basic knowledge in the biological and behavioural sciences is requisite to the application of principles and concepts from those sciences to nursing. Without a theoretical base, discussion of ethical issues may be merely sharing of opinions. Two basic theoretical approaches are (1) teleological, which is goal-directed or consequence-oriented, and (2) deontological, which is duty-oriented or focused on rules. Kluge (1992) identifies the difference between the two approaches "in the sorts of considerations they find relevant in reaching their conclusions" (p. 17). The teleological approach focuses on the anticipated outcome of actions, whereas "the deontological approach concentrates on balancing rights and duties . . . and considers them independently of outcome considerations" (Kluge, 1992, p. 17).

Although it is not feasible to provide a theoretical base for ethical decision making in this context, basic concepts of ethics can be identified. They include (1) *personhood,* of which self-awareness is a basic quality (Storch, 1982); (2) *autonomy,* which implies not only freedom to decide and to act but also to acknowledge and respect the dignity and autonomy of others (Francoeur, 1983); however, a health professional "has the obligation to intervene if the patient's choice is not in his/her best interests, particularly when there is reason to believe that the benefit is very great and harm would be significant" (Fry as interpreted by Reid, 1992, p. 26); (3) *veracity,* which includes obligation to tell the truth and to use good judgement in determining what the patient wants to know or can withstand; (4) *paternalism,* which refers to restricting the rights of an individual without his/her consent with the justification of trying to do good, such as not telling a person about his/her diagnosis and condition because of a poor prognosis; (5) *confidentiality,* which must be maintained but balanced against the rights of others, including society (Francoeur, 1983); (6) *beneficence,* or doing what is best for an individual while balancing the risks and benefits in a given situation; (7) *nonmaleficence,* or not inflicting intentional harm or risk of harm and preventing evil or harm whenever possible; and (8) *justice,* which pertains to ensuring that individuals get what they deserve according to individual need, worth, and merit and to enforcing the concept of distributive justice, which "has to do with the distribution of good and evil, of burdens and benefits in any society when resources are limited" (Davis and Aroskar, 1983, p. 45). The question of justice is an ethical dilemma frequently encountered today with cutbacks in funding and layoff of nurses, which may require nurses to make difficult decisions about apportioning care when all needs cannot be met.

Knowledge of basic ethical concepts is necessary for nurses to be able to address the increasingly complex issues encountered daily in practice settings. Although there is a tendency to consider only the ethical dilemmas faced in acute care settings, the issues are different but equally complex for practitioners in long-term care settings and in the community due to increased longevity, early discharge from hospital, and the use of technologies in the home that previously were limited to acute care settings. Robillard et al (1989) point out that there has been little research on the ethical issues in primary care, although most health care is provided in primary care settings. Their study revealed that the issues are most frequently pragmatic, not dramatic, and are concerned with "patient self-determination, adequacy of care and professional responsibility, and distribution of resources" (Robillard et al, 1989, p. 9). Thus nurses practising in all types of health-care settings need a knowledge base in ethical concepts and principles, as well as support and expert resources to assist them in ensuring that basic human rights are recognized and respected.

■ An Overview of the Canadian Legal System

The origins of the Canadian legal system can be found in English common law and Roman law. Quebec provincial law is derived from Roman law, the basis of the latter being found in The Twelve Tables of Rome (450 BC), Justinian's Code (533 AD), and the Napoleonic Code of 1804 (Merryman, 1969). The roots of English common law began more recently with the Norman conquest of 1066 (Plucknett, 1956). The law sets the parameters for human activity by defining rules for judging the acceptability of individual and corporate behaviour. In a sense the law defines our culture by outlining how we may behave based on certain social values and by providing deterrents to deviance from acceptable behaviour. The institutions of the law in our society are the provincial legislatures and the Parliament of Canada, which are entrusted with the creation of law through the passage of acts; the police forces across the country whose mandate is the enforcement of the law; the courts as the arbitrators of disputes; and the prisons, which are responsible for applying punishments for breaking the law.

The major types of law are case law and enacted law. The traditions of English common law are such that case law is dominant, whereas in the Roman civil law tradition, enacted law is the primary form of law that is mainly statutory. In Canada, these two traditions survive with the two founding nations. The Quebec civil code is based on the Roman tradition, while in the rest of Canada, the traditions of English common law prevail. According to Dais (1973), enacted law has become more important in areas where the traditions of common law are the primary form of the law. However, these usually do not extend to codes such as those customary under Roman traditions that incorporate detailed descriptions of daily life.

Although the courts are often thought of as the major component of the judicial system, other important components include the legal profession and the adversary system. The major types of law include civil or private law, which incorporates contract, tort, and property law, while public law includes constitutional, administrative, and criminal law. International law involves both of these types of law. Where the law is concerned with individuals, it is thought of as private law, while where it is concerned with governments, it falls within public law (Dais, 1973). In Canada, jury trials are primarily reserved for criminal cases and are used for very few civil cases. This is different from the United States where the traditions of English common law also prevail and where jury trials are more often used in civil cases. Because of the considerable expenses associated with jury trials, the Canadian approach tends to be less costly.

■ Legal Responsibilities of Nurses

Nurses have important legal obligations to the public as professionals who have close relationships with people. As health care has changed, so have nurses' responsibilities towards their clients. In tertiary care settings, nurses have become responsible for procedures that are highly technical and with which considerably greater risk is involved than was true in the past. Even in community settings this holds true in many situations. Thus on a daily basis, nurses have more chance of violating the rights of others, simply because of the nature of the acts for which they have become responsible. Just as for physicians and other health professionals, the public expects that nurses will practise safely and competently according to the ethical principles that have been previously identified. When cases are in dispute, the concept of the provision of a reasonable standard of care is what courts look to in terms of deciding whether a particular nurse acted prudently in a particular situation.

■ Clients' Rights and Nurses' Obligations in Health Care

Basic Human Rights in Health Care

Basic human rights in health care, which are recognized increasingly today, are the right to be informed, the right to be respected, and the right to self-determination. Each has great implications for ethical decision making and the responsibility of health professionals to protect rights. These rights also cause debate over ethical issues and are the bases for confrontation between nurses and physicians. For example, there may be differences of opinion between nurses and physicians about the meaning of being informed and whose responsibility it is to inform the individual and family. A confrontation may occur when information is withheld by a physician who believes this is in the best interest of the patient when the nurse believes that the patient should be informed and is asked directly for such information. The right to be informed has increased the need for obtaining informed consent before medical interventions are instituted and before patients are asked to participate in research. Until the 1970s, there was no expectation or requirement for obtaining informed consent for participation in research, and people were sometimes exploited. For example, in an experiment at the Allen Memorial Institute in Montreal in the late 1940s, patients were administered mind-altering drugs, such as lysergic acid diethylamide (LSD), which had far-reaching effects, and recompense was sought and obtained through legal action in the 1980s.

The right to be respected has great implications for approaches to patients and is interrelated with the right to be informed. Providing an interpretation of care and explaining medical conditions in understandable language are two methods of showing respect for an individual. Respect also has implications for confidentiality, which has been a problem in terms of information shared among health professionals. Although nurses and physicians may respect confidentiality to the point of not sharing information with persons outside the health professions, there is a tendency to share information openly in discussions where it can be overheard. Confidentiality also requires that written records be carefully protected, which has great implications for protecting rights with the expanding use of computers for storage and retrieval of patient data.

The right to self-determination implies that individuals or families have the right to make decisions about matters that affect their health and their lives. Ensuring that this right is protected is complex; for example, it involves deciding if an individual is capable of making decisions and if not, who should be involved in the decision making. Making decisions about matters that affect a patient's health and life involves giving people the opportunity to decide not to have treatment recommended by a physician. This is a difficult situation for health professionals because they are faced with an individual refusing treatment that they believe is best for that individual. There may be circumstances in which not consenting to the treatment is logical in view of the individual's prognosis and desire not to undergo adverse side effects known to result from some treatments, such as cancer therapy when the disease has progressed beyond redemption. On the other hand, some individuals choose to have treatment almost to the end, even if there is no hope of cure or remission.

Self-determination is not limited to life and death matters; it also involves decisions about life-styles. For example, individuals make decisions to continue with lifestyles and behaviour patterns that are known to be detrimental to their health and well-being, such as smoking, overeating, excessive drinking, refusing to wear seat belts, and engaging in sexual relations with people likely to be carriers of the acquired immunodeficiency virus. Although efforts to educate the public about the hazards of such habits are achieving successes, many persons still choose to do things that are harmful to their health.

Code of Ethics

A code of ethics is one of the characteristics of a profession. It is defined by the profession through the professional association and is designed to inform members of that profession and society about the profession's expectations in ethical matters. For many years, physicians have taken the Hippocratic Oath on graduating from medical school. Although it provides some ethical direction, it also can be interpreted as committing the physician to save or prolong life at any cost. This is one of the factors leading to stressful interprofessional relationships when physicians consider it their responsibility to decide about prolonging life, and nurses believe the individual and/or family should be involved in making decisions that affect their lives.

> **A VALUE AND RESULTING OBLIGATIONS FOR NURSES**
>
> **Value IV ... Dignity of Clients**
>
> The nurse is guided by consideration for the dignity of clients.
>
> **Obligations**
>
> 1. Nursing care must be done with consideration for the personal modesty of clients.
> 2. A nurse's conduct at all times should acknowledge the client as a person. For example, discussion of care in the presence of the client should actively involve or include that client.
> 3. Nurses have a responsibility to intervene when other participants in the health care system fail to respect any aspect of client dignity.
> 4. As ways of dealing with death and the dying process change, nursing is challenged to find new ways to preserve human values, autonomy and dignity. In assisting the dying clients, measures must be taken to afford the clients as much comfort, dignity and freedom from anxiety and pain as possible. Special consideration must be given to the need of the client's family or significant others to cope with their loss.

From Canadian Nurses Association. (1991). *Code of ethics for nursing.* Ottawa: The Association, p. 7.

In 1955 the Canadian Nurses Association (CNA) adopted the code of ethics developed in 1953 by the International Council of Nurses (ICN) and replaced in 1973 by the *ICN Code for Nurses—Ethical Concepts Applied to Nursing,* to guide Canadian nurses in ethical decision making. In 1978 the CNA membership decided to make the development of a national code of ethics a priority; the first *CNA Code of Ethics for Nursing* was approved in 1980. It was revised in 1985 and again in 1991 based on input from nurses using it in practice and was distributed to all CNA members with *The Canadian Nurse,* CNA's official journal received monthly by members.

This Code expresses and seeks to clarify the obligation of nurses to use their knowledge and skills for the benefit of others, to minimize harm, to respect client autonomy and to provide fair and just care for their clients. For those entering the profession, this Code identifies the basic moral commitments of nursing and may serve as a source of education and reflection. For those within the profession, the Code also serves as a basis for self-evaluation and for peer review. For those outside the profession, this Code may serve to establish expectations for the ethical conduct of nurses (CNA, November 1991, p. ii).

The Code presents values, or broad ideals, and obligations arising from each value that provide direction in particular circumstances. Some values pertain to clients or patients; other values are concerned with nursing roles and relationships. An example of a value and the obligations deriving therefrom is shown in the box above.

Although codes of ethics may or may not be part of statutory regulations, in most provinces there is a statutory requirement within the Act governing the nursing profession, which mandates that nurses uphold ethical standards as defined by the nursing profession. This means that not only are individual nurses expected to uphold the precepts contained in codes of ethics, but also hold colleagues accountable for adhering to them. Thus codes of ethics contain statements of moral accountability, which "provide an enforceable standard of minimally decent conduct that allows the profession to discipline those who clearly fall below the standard . . . (and indicate) some of the ethical considerations professionals must take into account in deciding on conduct" (Benjamin and Curtis, 1986, p. 6).

Because of the complexity of the ethical dilemmas nurses confront today, they need more than a code of ethics. Storch (1982) believes that at least four conditions are necessary for ethical decision making: (1) desire and commitment to do what is right and good; (2) knowledge of relevant facts of the particular situation; (3) clarity of thought, rather than emotionalism, in dealing with the facts; and (4) some understanding of basic principles or concepts of ethics. In recent years, nurses and other health professionals have recognized the importance of examining and clarifying values that may influence their actions and of becoming more sensitive to the values of their patients. Rather than prescribing a set of values, values clarification strategies are being used increasingly in both nursing education programs and continuing education programs for practising nurses.

The Right to Make Choices in Relation to Death

Death and dying give rise to many ethical issues and dilemmas. Davis and Aroskar (1983) identify three issues: (1) possible interventions by health professionals, such as resuscitation and passive euthanasia; (2) possible interventions by the family or significant others, such as helping a terminally ill person to hasten death and end suffering; and (3) possible interventions by the afflicted person, such as suicide, use of a living will, and claiming a right to die.

The word, *euthanasia,* is derived from Greek meaning good or pleasant death. Is death ever preferable to life? That question is difficult to answer. One must consider each specific situation and distinguish it from the interests and values of the care provider and the institution. Some think that euthanasia should be considered only for those who can ask to die, which would eliminate newborns, infants, and individuals kept alive by machines and unable to speak for themselves. Others believe that in certain circumstances some severely deformed newborns should be allowed to die by withdrawing or withholding treatments and that the decision should be made by the parents and their professional advisors, who are usually physicians (Duff and Campbell, 1973; McCormick, 1974; Shaw, 1973).

Passive euthanasia, or "letting someone die," may be done by not initiating treatment, with or without consent of the individual. These measures, although used in some hospitals, are still morally controversial. Active euthanasia is providing an individual with the means to end life or directly bringing about the individual's death with or without consent (Brody, 1976). How does the concept of protecting human rights fit into euthanasia? Does a person ever have the right to die? Can one refuse life-saving treatment? Is lack of clear-cut policies and guidelines to help health professionals in addressing such complex questions a reflection of there being no right or wrong answer? Some believe that death should never be hastened; others believe that a person whose death is imminent should be allowed to die to relieve pain and suffering and that the right to refuse treatment should be respected. Some fear that if euthanasia as a kindly act—beneficent euthanasia—can be morally justified, euthanasia for other purposes may also be justified and practised (Dyck, 1975).

■ Nurses' Actions Under the Law

Consent to Nursing Care

The right to be free from interference is a fundamental human right. Because nursing in some settings may involve a great deal of touching of others, it is important to recognize that the nurse must obtain consent from the client before touching occurs. Battery is a tort that involves intentional touching of another person, and there is no requirement that the person be injured as a result of the touching. In practice, clients rarely bring legal proceedings if there has not been serious harm as a result of touching. However, it is important that ever nurse be very careful to explain nursing procedures to clients and to obtain consent prior to initiating a procedure. Effective communication between nurses and clients is vital, and explaining and obtaining the patient's permission to carry out procedures is an essential part of this communication.

Consent to care may be expressed, implied, or inferred. In the past, nurses have often relied on implied consent for procedures. However, Philpott (1985) has stated that in the absence of emergency conditions or in the case of procedures involving considerable risk, it is unwise to rely on implied consent. The following six elements must be present in legal consent:

1. The consent must be genuine and voluntary.
2. The procedure must not be an illegal procedure.
3. The consent must authorize the particular performer of the treatment or care.
4. The consenter must have legal capacity to consent.
5. The consenter must have the necessary mental competency to consent.
6. The consenter must be informed (p. 57).

Even though such issues as age, health and mental status of clients may make it difficult for the nurse to obtain informed consent, it is nonetheless essential to do so in the appropriate way for the circumstances present in each situation.

Confidentiality

Nurses often think of confidentiality exclusively as an ethical issue. It is important to understand that the client's right to confidentiality is embedded in the provincial hospital acts. However, acts regulating nursing also specify the nurse's professional responsibility to maintain client confidentiality. A nurse who fails to carry out this responsibility may be subject to allegations of professional misconduct. The provinces of Quebec, British Columbia, Manitoba, and Saskatchewan also protect the right of privacy by statutes providing for this. Provinces where the only references to privacy are in the hospital acts do not provide the same level of protection. Section 7 of *The Charter of Rights and Freedoms* contains an area that has not yet been explored and may be used in future challenges made under the charter: "Everyone has the right to life, liberty and security of the person and the right not to be deprived thereof except in accordance with the principles of fundamental justice" (p. 11).

There are certain exceptions to the responsibility to maintain confidentiality. These include situations in which the client gives consent to disclose personal information to those not named in the provincial hospital act, statutory provisions for reporting certain diseases and child abuse to certain health and social agencies, and court orders for the purpose of obtaining health records for the use of plaintiffs or defendants in trials. Although the client's right to view personal health records has been a controversial issue in the past for those pursuing legal action against a health care agency or its employees, there is increasing recognition that clients have a right to see their records. It is likely that as new legislation on confidentiality is developed, this right will be recognized.

Collaboration with Physicians

Nurses work in close collaboration with physicians and, in cases where physicians have communicated their wishes in relation to a patient's treatment to nurses over the telephone, occasional misunderstandings have occurred. In any situation where written directions for treatment are not made at the time directions are given, the potential for misinterpretation exists. Where telephone orders are acceptable within a health care agency, a nurse may be liable if there is later disagreement with a physician over the orders. The increasing complexity of health care means that risks for nurses are also increasing. If telephone orders are allowable in the health care agency, there should be a system for contemporaneous external validation of the orders to enhance safety for the client and to ensure that the nurse is not subject to unwarranted risk. This could take the form of taping and transcription of telephone orders or of having the order validated by a second nurse at the time it is given.

Nursing Documentation

The Supreme Court of Canada declared that nurses' notes were admissible in court in 1970 (*Ares v Venner*, 1970). This attests to the importance of nurses' records of the care provided to and progress made by clients in their care and means that nurses' notes could serve to support cases for or against nurses, physicians or hospitals. The importance of "the virtues of accuracy, legibility, brevity practised faithfully by the nurse" in enhancing the value of nursing documentation to the care of the client has been underscored by Ross (1973, p. 102). In the event of "unusual occurrence" or "incident reports" that are most often written by nurses, the importance of a "cool, dispassionate, and thoughtful" approach to making a "factual, concise and totally objective" record of the event is supported by the fact that incident records could be introduced as evidence to support or defend a damage claim (Ross, 1973, p. 102-103).

Problems with nurses' notes have frequently been the subject of criticism in court records of proceedings, thus underscoring the importance of the principles of recording referred to above. Failure to record events immediately after they have happened can be a serious matter because of the fact that individuals are likely to forget details which might be very important in a particular situation if time elapses between the time the event happened and the time it was described in a written record. Recording of care by someone other than the nurse who provided the care also casts doubt on the validity of the record. Care provided but not recorded is difficult to verify. The fact that cases often come to trial long after the events in dispute occurred makes it difficult for principals to remember critical details in such situations. The importance of a clear, comprehensive, and detailed written record cannot be underestimated. This is not to say that nurses should spend their time recording everything done for clients. Many believe that this is wasteful both in terms of the highly skilled professional nurse and unnecessary. Charting by exception, a method by which unusual occurrences and reactions only are recorded, is becoming more common in health care agencies. It is evident that good judgement and considerable discretion, however, must be used in determining what should and should not be recorded.

With the advent of computerization in hospitals and other health agencies where nurses are employed, new issues are emerging. Legibility of records is no longer a problem, but issues related to the nature and quality of the recording continue to be important. Program parameters can be set so that it is not possible to alter the time notation on the record and to eliminate additions to the text of a record written at an earlier time. Although signatures may not be possible, identifying codes for each user may help to ensure that the identify of the writer is known. Confidentiality of computerized records is also a potential problem since more people may have access to the record than was the case before computerization. In the development of appropriate systems for client records, providing access only to those with a need to do so is an important issue. Storage of records in a computerized file rather than in hard copy will minimize the space required to store large numbers of records and potentially facilitate prompt access to a client's previous health history.

Negligence

Negligence or that which a reasonable and prudent nurse would or would not do in particular health care circumstances is the basis for most lawsuits against health professionals. Philpott has listed the following conditions that must be present for a defendant to be held liable for damages in court:

1. The presence of a duty of care by the defendant to the plaintiff.
2. The defendant's conduct must constitute a breach of that duty of care; i.e., must have failed to comply with the required standard of care.
3. The plaintiff must have suffered an injury.
4. The negligent conduct must have been the proximate cause of the injury.
5. There must not have been contributory negligence on the part of the plaintiff and he must not have voluntarily assumed the risk (1985, p. 25).

How the reasonable and prudent nurse would have acted in a similar situation is established by courts in a number of ways. These include articles and books by nursing authors documenting the acceptability or lack of acceptability of certain practices, nursing practice standards developed by national and provincial professional nursing organizations, records of curriculum content in schools of nursing, and testimony by expert nurse witnesses. A nurse whose conduct is being scrutinized in court may expect that areas of interest to legal counsel will be the quality of practice, educational background, experience, and efforts to maintain knowledge and competence on an ongoing basis. In one important case, a nurse was found negligent after it was established that the nurse, who had worked in a physician's office in Alberta for 22 years, had failed to take any continuing education courses since the year after she had graduated, some 40 years before (*Dowey v Rothwell*, 1974).

Canadian Nurses Protective Society

It is clearly evident that a primary concern for nurses should be to maintain a high level of competence in nursing practice, excellent communication with clients, and an awareness of the risks involved in performing nursing procedures. Nurses also must have some knowledge of the law, legal processes, the judicial system, the rights of their clients, and their own responsibilities. The Canadian Nurses Protective Society (CNPS) was established by the Canadian Nurses Association in 1988. Up to this time, the provincial/territorial nursing associations had contracted with insurance firms for professional liability insurance that members obtained as a component of their membership in these associations. Associations perceived a need to develop an organization managed by the profession to minimize escalating costs of obtaining professional liability insurance on a province-by-province basis through insurance firms. The CNPS is a nonprofit organization offering professional liability insurance and is purchased by ten of the twelve provincial/territorial associations on behalf of their members (all provincial/territorial associations except British Columbia and Quebec). The CNPS offers advice about professional liability to nurses from 0845 to 1630 hours Monday to Friday EST. Nurses may call CNPS about any situation with ethical/legal implications in which they have personal involvement or knowledge by calling a toll-free telephone number (1-800-267-3390) outside Ottawa or 237-2133 in Ottawa. Nurses may speak with a nurse-lawyer who will give immediate advice and assistance about steps to take in documenting an unusual occurrence, understanding legal processes, and in referring nurses to experienced legal counsel.

■ Ethical Dilemmas in Health Care

Do Not Resuscitate Orders

Practising nurses are keenly aware of the ethical dilemmas they face in relation to "do not resuscitate" (DNR) or "no code" orders. If there is no written DNR order and a patient arrests, is the nurse expected to "code" the patient? Who is, or should be, involved in making such a decision? Are there, or should there be, differences in DNR policies in long-term care institutions versus acute-care settings? The development of guidelines for resuscitation has been encouraged through a joint effort of the Canadian Medical Association (CMA), Canadian Nurses Association (CNA), Canadian Hospital Association (CHA), and Canadian Bar Association (CBA), which resulted in a "Joint Statement on Terminal Illness" published in 1984 in *The Canadian Nurse* (1984). The guidelines have been used in formulating policy and procedure for institutions; however, they address only patients who are terminally ill and do not address such issues as chronic illness and age. Toth (1991, p. 5) states unequivocally that CPR should not be performed "on a patient for whom such an intervention would prolong the dying process rather than extend life," and that "strong consideration should be given to a policy that would make CPR the exception rather than the rule in long-term care institutions." The University of Alberta Hospitals' policy for "No CPR Order" reflects Toth's thinking in its rationale, stating: "CPR should not be attempted in cases in which such an intervention is not in the best interests of the patient. CPR performed for inappropriate indications may prolong the dying process rather than extend life and may lead to futile suffering of patients" (August 12, 1991). The rationale states further that health-care professionals are responsible for keeping informed about research findings "following attempted CPR in different age groups and disease states" so decisions about CPR are research-based. Although it is the physician's responsibility to write a DNR order and also convey the meaning of it to the nursing staff, there should be opportunity for nursing input into the development of such guidelines. Davis and Aroskar (1983, p. 149) point out that "nurses are in a key position to notify the physician if the patient's condition changes, which change would indicate that the orders may need reassessment." This reinforces the need for careful nursing assessment and clear communication with physicians and the need for flexibility and wise judgment in applying orders based on changes in the patient's condition.

The policy indicates the importance of discussing the DNR order with the patient, guardian and family and also recording this in the progress notes; however, the literature raises questions about the extent to which patients are involved in such decisions. In a study of older adults in an acute-care and long-term care setting, Godkin (1992) found that most of the patients had limited knowledge of CPR and its possible outcomes and that this knowledge was gained primarily through television in which most of the attempts to resuscitate were successful. The question of CPR had not been discussed by a physician with the majority, and most had not discussed their wishes regarding care with anyone. Nonetheless, if given an opportunity, 85% would have chosen to be involved in deciding whether to have CPR, and 75% "hoped that their physician would inform them if they thought that CPR would be of no benefit to them" (Godkin, 1992, p. 114). Most of the patients favoured a collaborative approach to decisions about CPR, involving physicians, themselves, nurses, and family members. Most DNR policies in hospitals pertain to terminally ill patients only. Godkin (1992) suggests that such policies be made known so that every individual understands that current policy requires that CPR be performed on other patients unless a DNR order is recorded on the chart. This would require that the issue be addressed which could reduce the dilemmas faced by families and staff regarding CPR, reduce costs of giving CPR that was not desired by the patients, and prevent the situation of patients being unable to participate in the decision by the time any discussion is initiated.

Although autonomous decision making by the patients is highly valued by both nurses and physicians, recent research shows that frequently the patient is not involved in the decision where participation is possible (Bedell and Delbanco, 1984; Bedell, Pelle, Maher, and Cleary, 1986; Evans and Brody, 1985; Savage, Cullen, Kirchhoff, Pugh, and Foreman, 1987). Bedell and Delbanco (1984) surveyed 154 physicians whose patients had been resuscitated and found that only 19% of the patients had discussed resuscitation with the physician before cardiac arrest occurred. They also found that 33% of the families had been consulted about resuscitation beforehand, but patients' competency to be involved in the decision had not been addressed. Youngner (1987) suggests some possible reasons physicians may not discuss resuscitation with their patients: lack of awareness; pressure of time; discomfort about discussing such matters; and/or the paternalistic attitude of doing what the physician feels is best for the patient. Such reactions fail to support the patient's right to self-determination and autonomy.

In a study of DNR policies and end-of-life decisions in acute care settings in Alberta, Wilson (1993) found that 73% of the 135 accredited health-care facilities had a written DNR policy. Most had been developed in the 1990s to optimize decision making and involve the patient in the process; however, these purposes had not been achieved in general. In-depth surveys of four of the facilities indicated that DNR policies were not commonly followed and that in almost one-third of instances they were not implemented at all. Problems generally arose from late decision making that excluded the patient from end-of-life decisions. Hence, DNR policies seems to have limited effect on practice. Wilson (1993) identifies the need for internal assessment to determine the extent to which nurses and physicians are knowledgeable about the DNR policy. Further, she believes that if the policy is retained, adherence should be emphasized since "lack of adherence to organizational policy places health-care facilities in legal and ethical jeopardy" (p. 127). She suggests additional education about policies and perhaps designating a separate DNR chart form to improve recording and help to guide decision making about DNR.

Wilson (1993) also found that no-CPR decisions were usually made late and hence, did not create an ethical or legal dilemma for health professionals or family members "as everything possible appeared to have been done to restore health and prevent death" (p. 129). She noted that it was common practice for health professionals to use at least one life-sustaining technology, such as oxygen and/or intravenous therapy, to promote comfort during the end-stage dying process. Questioning whether comfort was always the outcome, Wilson (1993) identifies the need for research to substantiate or refute whether such measures promote comfort or just extend the dying process.

Yarling and McElmurry (1983) propose authorizing both the responsible physician and the responsible nurse to write DNR orders, depending on the situation. Although this may seem like an onerous responsibility for the nurse, is it any greater than having to perform CPR when the nurse knows that the patient does not want it? While it seems unlikely that nurses will be granted such a privilege, it is important that nurses and physicians have mechanisms to discuss such questions and differences of opinion. Also, it is important that patients have opportunity to participate in making such profound decisions in advance of the critical occurrence, such as provided by advance directives.

Advance Directives

In recent years much attention has been given to developing directives in advance to serve as guidelines for health practitioners and family members when an individual is no longer capable of making decisions. A report, *Advance Directives and Substitute Decision-Making in Personal Care*, published in March 1993 by the Alberta Law Reform Institute and the Health Law Institute, recommends that:

> legislation be introduced to enable individuals to execute a health care directive, in which they can (1) appoint someone as their health care agent, who will have authority to make health care decisions on their behalf in the event of their being incapable of making those decisions personally; (2) identify anyone whom they do not wish to act as their health care proxy; and (3) provide instructions and information concerning future health care decisions (Alberta Law Reform Institute, March 1993, p. 94).

Similar legal developments have taken place, or are in process, in Manitoba, Ontario, Newfoundland, British Columbia, and Saskatchewan. Storch and Dossetor (1994) found overwhelming support for the concept of advance health care directives in a survey of Edmonton residents. Similarly, strong support for it was found by Hughes and Singer (1992) in their survey of 1000 family physicians in Ontario; however, their findings also revealed that most respondents rarely discuss the idea with their patients.

Advance directives may be prepared in the form of a living will that enables individuals to indicate in advance whether they want "heroic or extraordinary measures" in the event they are unable to make known their wishes. This approach was rejected by the Alberta Law Reform Institute and Health Law Institute because of problems of interpretation with the use of such vague terms as "heroic" and "extraordinary" measures. For example, do they refer to CPR only, or do they include tube feeding and other measures designed to prolong life? They also rejected the durable power of attorney approach that "enables an individual, while mentally competent, to appoint someone who will have the authority to make health care decisions on the donor's behalf once the donor becomes mentally incapable of making these decisions" (Joint Report, 1993, p. 7). Rather, their approach is to legalize the concept of health care directives so individuals can have control over who will make decisions on their behalf when they are unable to do so and also have some control over the content of decisions by including specific instruction in the directive, if desired.

If advance directives are enacted by the Alberta legislature, Wilson (1993) emphasizes the need for health-care facilities to review, and perhaps revise, their DNR policy to change the method in which life support preferences are determined and used in decision making about care. Even if such legislation is not enacted, Wilson's findings indicate a need for action to enhance patient self-determination.

Flarey (1991, p. 19) identifies three major advantages for use of advance directives: (1) to ensure that one's predetermined wishes are followed; (2) to help family members in making complex decisions; and (3) to provide guidance to health professionals regarding the individual's wishes in such circumstances. Despite these advantages, their use will depend on the extent to which health-care agencies develop and implement such policies and inquire of patients whether they have developed an advance directive. Nurses can play an important role in ensuring that these goals are attained in their work settings by gaining representation on ethics committees and other policy-making bodies on advance directives, and by educating colleagues and the public about individual rights to self-determination.

Issues in Childbearing

A major ethical issue pertaining to childbearing is abortion. The issue is "the status of the fetus as a member of the human species when the existence of the fetus poses a threat to the physical, psychological or social well-being of a pregnant woman and/or other family members" (Curtin, 1982, p. 240). Anti-abortionists claim that the personhood of the fetus is being denied, whereas pro-abortionists maintain that the woman's right to self-determination cannot be denied. They emphasize the burden imposed on society by an unwanted pregnancy and possible outcomes for the welfare of the child in the future. Between the two extremes are those who favour abortions depending on circumstances surrounding the pregnancy, such as rape and incest.

The question of abortion may present problems for the individual nurse who is expected to participate in the care of patients having an abortion. The nurse is responsible, legally and morally, for ensuring that patients' needs are met and that patients are not neglected because of differing values (Curtin, 1982). It is important that nurses know the agency's policies about such participation before accepting a position. Health-care agencies must have clearly defined policies that can be communicated to potential employees and referred to when situations arise that present an ethical dilemma to staff members.

The Supreme Court of Canada's decision, made in 1988, endorses women's rights to self-determination in relation to abortion. This has been challenged many times, but the challenges have not been supported. For example, Bill C43 passed in 1990 by the House of Commons, would permit abortion only if a continued pregnancy would jeopardize the woman's physical or mental health, as diagnosed by one physician only. Physicians adamantly opposed this change because of the possibility of criminal charges against them and because they would be required to provide pre-abortion and post-abortion counseling. Bill C-43 was struck down; thus the Supreme Court's decision still prevails.

Allocation of Health-Care Resources and Rationing of Health Care

Ethical issues pertaining to allocation of health-care resources may be encountered at several levels. At the government level, public policies are established that determine what type of health care can be provided. Nurses and other health professionals have a responsibility to exercise their prerogatives and communicate with legislators to influence these policies. For example, as a result of a government's decision not to require seat belt use by law, a considerable portion of the health-care dollar is spent on persons involved in automobile accidents.

Policies that influence the use of health-care resources are also established at the institutional level. Too often, nurses have little influence on such policies, and they need to take action to affect decision making and priority setting. Decisions to develop programs are often made without adequate consideration of the implications for nursing practice; medical programs, such as heart transplants and joint replacements, have a great impact on the need for nursing care and could affect nurses' ability to respond to the demands placed on them. At the unit level, nurses have to delineate problems that result from new programs and provide data that will facilitate a reasoned decision, although values and emotions often enter into these decisions. Fortunately, nurses have become more vocal in expressing their concerns and in providing facts that can influence decision making, rather than merely responding to the decisions made by the physicians and hospital administrators.

Is it ethically and morally right to support activities that may jeopardize the patient or result in unequal or unfair distribution of resources among different programs within a health-care institution? Who determines the priorities in allocating resources, and what facts are considered? With the increasing proportion of older persons in Canada and other developed countries, the question of age may influence decisions even with the lobbying power seniors have developed. Many disadvantaged groups, such as the physically handicapped, the retarded, the poor, and ethnic minorities, may also be exploited by such decisions.

Other factors that influence allocation of resources in health-care legislation include consumer unrest and the patients' rights movement. Davis and Aroskar (1983, p. 26) believe that "health care policy cannot be the monopoly of providers any more than scientists should have the only say on biomedical research." Reasons for such a position are possible conflicts of interest; the large amount of taxes used to provide health care; nonmedical dimensions of health problems that may be critical aspects; and that "individual liberty and autonomy extend not only into the political arena but also into health care" (Davis and Aroskar, 1983, p. 206). Although nurses, individually and collectively have become more involved in influencing public policy through lobbying and working effectively with consumers and providers of care, their involvement needs to be increased. In addition to responding to particular issues, the professional organizations can work to influence public policy about allocation of health-care resources.

Expenditures for health care as a percentage of Gross Domestic Product have been slowly rising over the past four decades since the advent of national health insurance in 1957. The practice of deficit budgeting adopted by the federal government in the 1970s and by provincial governments in the 1980s led by 1994 to large accumulated debt attributable to provincial and national governments. At 9.9% of Gross Domestic Product in 1991, national expenditures for health care became obvious targets for cuts and downsizing of health programs (Health Canada, 1994). In such a climate, concern and scrutiny of all health expenditures has occurred and governments are increasingly slashing spending in all areas. However, the legacy of federal government failure to defend the provisions of the Canada Health Act since 1984 and of escalating expenditures for health provincially and federally, has been a questioning of the viability of the five basic principles of the Canada Health Act. Within certain provinces, facility fees for payments to physicians for services received in private health care establishments have been permitted, thus undermining the public administration principle and the prohibiting of user fee charges of the Canada Health Act.

Although there has always been rationing of health care in the Canadian health system, it has not been systematically applied. The development of criteria for the admission of clients to certain treatment programs such as kidney, heart, or liver transplant programs has been carried out in health care agencies for a considerable period of time, primarily because the costs of such services are high and the attempt has been to use resources in the most appropriate manner to benefit citizens. Some health professionals may have failed to fully inform clients about treatment options, believing the course of action suggested to be the most important in the particular situation. In a society where health care consumers are more knowledgeable and where the professional has an ethical and legal duty to make full knowledge of treatment and care possible available to clients and their families, more attention is being focused on the need to make rational choices about the provision of care balanced by reasonable access to care of a comprehensive nature on a universal basis to all qualified residents of Canada. In other areas, physicians, nurses, and other health professionals have found themselves in situations where they were prolonging death rather than preserving life; increasingly, society is trying to come to grips with some of these situations. Models of rationing of care in the public system of medicare for those over 65 years of age in the United States are increasingly being discussed in Canada in terms of their applicability to or appropriateness in the Canadian context. Issues in rationing of care are likely to continue over the next decade as the health system undergoes major restructuring and reform.

■ Strategies for Addressing Ethical Dilemmas in Practice

The number and variety of ethical dilemmas that nurses encounter in practice have increased because of advancements in scientific knowledge and development of technologies. Nurses and physicians often become embroiled in ethical dilemmas in which opinions differ, leading to decreased communication and failure to work together in the interests of patients. These results can be detrimental to patient care and to the mental health and well-being of nursing staff, particularly in intensive care units, where nurses and physicians may disagree on life and death decisions, on approaches to care, and on setting priorities.

Some health-care agencies address these dilemmas through an ethics committee, which is called on an ad hoc basis to address dilemmas presented by nurses or physicians. In some large teaching hospitals an ethicist is employed to provide expert assistance and guidance. At the Montreal General Hospital, Dr. David Roy, an internationally renowned physician-ethicist, has been helping nursing and medical staff address complex issues for many years. Institutional ethics committees are not a new venture in Canadian hospitals. The Canadian Hospital Association issued a policy statement recommending them in 1966 (CHA, 1986). Avard, Griener and Langstaff (1985) conducted a survey to determine the extent to which they exist, their composition and modus operandi. Their findings revealed a great deal of variability in size, composition and function and that they were primarily advisory; however, the effectiveness of the committees was not ascertained. A second survey by Storch and Griener (1990) was designed to try to determine the effectiveness of committees in addressing the ethical problem in self-determination. The data revealed that the status of ethics committees in Canadian hospitals was very similar in 1994 to what it was in 1989. The most evident change was an increase from 18% to 58.3% of the hospitals having an ethics committee. Most respondents indicated that the committees serve primarily in an advisory capacity; however, it is not known whether such advice must be followed. To seek an answer to this question and others regarding the effectiveness of committees, a second phase of the study was undertaken through site visits to five selected hospitals for in-depth review, but the findings have not been reported to date.

A strategy of a preventive nature is to improve the teaching of ethics in nursing education by ensuring that ethics is an official part of the nursing curricula on the undergraduate and graduate levels and is taught by experts, not "left to chance" to be integrated into all teaching. Thompson and Thompson (1989) are advocates of this approach. They identify the goals of teaching ethics to professional students and professionals as: "to stimulate the moral imagination; recognize ethical issues; elicit a sense of moral obligation; develop analytical skills; and tolerate and reduce disagreements and ambiguity" (1989, p. 86). They recommend using case studies, as many textbooks on ethics include; however, there must be expert guidance available during the process of analyzing the ethical issues and dilemmas presented.

Since many practising nurses who face ethical dilemmas every day have not had the benefit of this education, discussion of ethics should be included in inservice education and continuing education. After nurses have learned the theoretical foundation of ethics, ongoing Bioethics Rounds can be organized for nurses and physicians. Bioethics Rounds are not intended to address ethical issues encountered in the care of a specific patient, but to provide opportunities for open discussion of ethical issues when the professionals involved can consider various viewpoints and are not facing a specific ethical issue requiring an immediate decision. Since 1987, this approach has been developed through the Bioethics Centre beginning by the University of Alberta and the University of Alberta Hospitals. The project, a result of a collaborative effort to address ethical dilemmas, has equal representation from medicine, nursing and philosophy through directors who plan and conduct Bioethics Rounds and are responsible for joint teaching in ethics for nursing and medical students. Such a collaborative approach facilitates addressing issues involving both professions so they are deliberated together, and collaborative decisions are reached that are in the best interests of the patients and health-care providers. This approach is based on the belief that collaboration in the delivery of health care is required to address complex ethical dilemmas; there are no right or wrong answers, but decisions must be made that will meet the needs of the consumers of health care.

In this chapter, a number of legal and ethical questions have been highlighted. Many more are addressed in books and journals for health professionals. The amount of literature on ethics has increased at a phenomenal rate in the past two decades, helping health professionals determine what actions to take in situations encountered in practice. Although there are no easy answers to ethical or legal questions, health professionals must have resources available, in the literature and through ethicists and legal experts, and they must use these resources in dealing with complex issues and dilemmas.

■ REFERENCES

Alberta Law Reform Institute. (1993). *Advance directives and substitute decision-making in personal health care*. A joint report of the Alberta Law Reform Institute and the Health Law Institute, Report No. 64, Edmonton, Alberta.

Ares v Venner. (1970). S.C.R., 14, D.L.R. (3d) 4 (S.C.C.), p. 608.

Avard, D., Griener, G., & Langstaff, J. (1985). Hospital ethics committees: Survey reveals characteristics. *Dimensions, 62*(2), 24-26.

Bedell, S. & Delbanco, T. (1984). Choices about cardiopulmonary resuscitation in the hospital. *New England Journal of Medicine, 300*, 310-317.

Bedell, S., Pelle, D., Maher, L, & Cleary, P. (1986). Do not resuscitate orders of critically ill patients in the hospital. *Journal of the American Medical Association, 256*, 2.

Benjamin, M. & Curtis, Jr. (1986). *Ethics in nursing*. (2nd ed). New York: Oxford University Press.

Brody, H. (1976). *Ethical decisions in medicine*. Boston: Little, Brown & Company.

Canadian Nurses Association. (1985). *Code of ethics for nursing*. Ottawa: The Association.

Canadian Nurses Association. (1991). *Code of ethics for nursing*. Ottawa: The Association.

Canadian Nurses Association, Canadian Medical Association and Canadian Hospital Association. (1984). Joint statement on terminal illness: A protocol for health professionals regarding resuscitative intervention for the terminally ill. *The Canadian Nurse, 80*(4), 24.

Curtin, L. L. (1982). Case study V: Abortion, privacy and conscience. In L. Curtin & M. J. Flaherty (Eds.), *Nursing ethics: Theories and pragmatics* (pp. 239-254). Bowie, MD: Robert J. Brady Company.

Curtin, L. L. (1985). Developing a professional ethic. *AARN Newsletter, 41*(10), 1, 3-6.

Dais, E. E. (1973). Canadian law: An overview. In S.R. Good & J.C. Kerr (Eds.), *Contemporary issues in Canadian law for nurses* (pp. 3-14). Toronto: Holt, Rinehart & Winston.

Davis, A. J. & Aroskar, M. A. (1983). *Ethical dilemmas and nursing practice* (2nd ed). Norwalk, CT: Appleton-Century-Crofts.

Dowey v Rothwell (1974). 5 W.W.R. 311.

Duff, R. S. & Campbell, A. G. M. (1973). Moral and ethical dilemmas in the special-care nursery. *New England Journal of Medicine, 289,* 89-894.

Dyck, A. J. (1975). Beneficent euthanasia and benemortasia: Alternative view of mercy. In M. Kohl (Ed.), *Beneficent euthanasia* (pp. 120-126). Buffalo, NY: Prometheus.

Evans, A. & Brody, B. (1985). The do not resuscitate order in teaching hospitals. *Journal of the American Medical Association, 253,* 15.

Flarey, D. (1991). Advanced directives: In search of self-determination. *Journal of Nursing Administration, 21*(11), 16-22.

Francoeur, R. T. (1983). *Biomedical ethics: A guide to decision making.* Toronto: John Wiley & Sons.

Fry, S. (1992). Ethics and accountability: A report by Doreen Reid. *AARN Newsletter, 48*(7), 25-26.

Godkin, M. D. (1992). Cardiopulmonary resuscitation: Knowledge, attitudes and opinions of older adults in acute care and long-term care settings. Unpublished master's thesis, University of Alberta Faculty of Nursing, Edmonton.

Grady, P. E. (1973). The law and nurses' notes. In S.R. Good & J.C. Kerr (Eds). *Contemporary issues in Canadian law for nurses* (pp. 127-129). Toronto: Holt, Rinehart & Winston.

Health Canada. (1994). Preliminary estimates of health expenditures in Canada. *Provincial-Territorial summary report, 1987-1991.* Ottawa: Health Information Division, Policy and Consultation Branch, Health Canada.

Hughes, D. L. & Singer, P. A. (1992). Family physicians' attitudes toward advance directives. *Canadian Medical Association Journal, 146*(11), 1937-1944.

International Council of Nurses. (1973). *ICN code for nurses—Ethical concepts applied to nursing.* Geneva, Switzerland: International Council of Nurses.

Kluge, E. W. (1992). *Biomedical ethics in a Canadian context.* Toronto: Prentice-Hall Canada, Inc.

McCormick, R. A. (1974). To save or let live: The dilemma of modern medicine. *Journal of the American Medical Association, 229,* 172-176.

Merryman, J. H. (1969). *The civil law tradition.* Palo Alto, CA: Stanford University Press.

Philpott, M. (1985). *Legal liability and the nursing process.* Toronto: W.B. Saunders.

Plucknett, T. F. T. (1956). *A concise history of the common law.* Boston: Little, Brown & Company.

Robillard, H. M., High, D. M., Sebastian, J. G., Pisaneschi, J. I., Perritt, L. J., & Mahler, D. M. (1989). Ethical issues in primary care: A survey of practitioners' perceptions. *Journal of Community Health, 14*(1), 9-17.

Ross, M. W. (1973). The nurse as an employee. In S. R. Good & J. C. Kerr (Eds.), *Contemporary issues in Canadian law for nurses* (pp. 95-106). Toronto: Holt, Rinehart & Winston.

Savage, T., Cullen, D., Kirchhoff, K., Pugh, E., & Foreman, M. (1987). Nurses' response to do not resuscitate orders in the neonatal intensive care unit. *Nursing Research, 36,* 6.

Shaw, A. (1973). Dilemmas of "informed consent" in children. *New England Journal of Medicine, 289,* 885-890.

Storch, J. L. (1982). *Patients' rights: Ethical and legal issues in health care and nursing.* Toronto: McGraw-Hill Ryerson.

Storch, J. L. & Griener, G. (June 1990). Ethics committees in Canadian hospitals: Report of 1989 survey. *The Bioethics Bulletin, 2*(2), 1-3. (Available from University of Alberta Division of Bioethics, Edmonton, Alberta.)

Storch, J. L. & Dossetor, J. B. (1994). Public attitudes toward end-of-life treatment decisions: Implications for nurse clinicians and nursing administrators. *Canadian Journal of Nursing Administration, 7*(3), 65-89.

Thompson, J. E. & Thompson, H. O. (1989). Teaching ethics to nursing students. *Nursing Outlook, 37*(2), 84-88.

Toth, E. (1991). Commentary on the national guidelines for no resuscitation orders. *The Bioethics Bulletin, 3*(3), 4-5. (Available from University of Alberta Division of Bioethics, Edmonton, Alberta.)

Wilson, D. M. (1993). The influences for do-not-resuscitate policies and end-of-life treatment or nontreatment decisions. Unpublished doctoral dissertation, University of Alberta, Edmonton.

Yarling, R. & McElmurry, B. (1983). Rethinking the nurse's role in do not resuscitate orders: A clinical policy proposal in nursing ethics. *Advances in Nursing Science, 5*(4), 1-12.

Youngner, S. J. (1987). DNR orders: No longer secret, but still a problem. *Hastings Center Report, 17*(1), 24-33.

6 Nursing Research as a Basis for Practice in Community Health Nursing

Jannetta MacPhail

In the past decade, nursing journals and conferences have emphasized increasingly clinical nursing research and the importance of strengthening the research base of nursing practice. Nursing research journals have been urged to include utilization of research findings as well as the usual reporting of research methods, findings and implications for practice. Indeed, in 1992 a new research journal, *Clinical Nursing Research*, was launched by Wood and Hayes at the University of Alberta with a clearly international perspective. What are the reasons for such an increased focus on clinical research and the application of research findings in nursing practice? What implications do the differences between community health nursing and other types of nursing practice have for the conduct of nursing research and the application of research findings? What are some of the facilitators and the deterrents of clinical research? What can practising nurses do to promote and support research? These are some of the questions to be addressed in this chapter.

■ Research-Based Nursing Practice

Research-based nursing practice is simply practice based on valid and reliable research findings from scientific investigation of nursing practice problems. Much of nursing practice today still is based on knowledge derived from trial-and-error experience or opinions and methods passed from generation to generation through books, articles, papers, conferences, workshops, and even through educational programs preparing students for entry to nursing practice. Nonetheless, an increasing number of nurses recognize the importance of research and research-based practice and are developing skills for critically evaluating research reports that are relevant for their practice.

The focus of nursing practise is helping people, whether sick or well, to attain, maintain, or regain their optimal level of health and functioning. Nursing practice includes health assessment and health promotion and encompasses a variety of strategies or interventions, such as teaching, anticipatory guidance, support, comfort measures, and compensatory measures. Compensatory activities are actions taken by the nurse to compensate for what the client cannot or will not do for himself or herself. They may include assisting with feeding to maintain nutritional status and elimination; assisting with ambulation to maintain circulation and joint and muscle function; and suctioning to maintain a clear airway. All such strategies are designed to enhance the individual's health-seeking behaviours; to stimulate avoidance of disease and disability; to promote maximum use of the person's own resources in coping with disease or dysfunction; and to help the person cope with family responsibilities and crises.

The nature of nursing practice requires nurses to study individual and group behaviour in relation to attaining, maintaining, and regaining health. To develop a scientific base for nursing practice, the focus of research is on people's behaviour pertaining to their motivation to be healthy, as well as their behaviour in coping with life crises. Life crises include such normal events as birth, developmental stages, and decline, as well as genetic failures, disease, and disability. Nursing research also may include behavioural responses to a wide variety of diagnostic and therapeutic interventions ordered by physicians. The feature that distinguishes nursing research from other research about human beings is the type of knowledge about people that nurses need and use in practice. Consequently, research to advance knowledge and improve practice focuses on people's behaviour in response to circumstances that require nursing actions and their behaviour in response to that action (Schlotfeldt, 1971).

Community health nursing differs from other types of nursing practice in that it focuses not only on individuals and families, but also on groups, aggregates, and the community as a whole. An aggregate is a subgroup within society whose members share one or more characteristics related to their health care needs. An example of such a subgroup might include children and youth who do not wear bicycle helmets and hence are at risk of head injury, or poor or neglected children who come to school hungry and unable to concentrate. Nonetheless, in actual practice community health nurses have focused on individuals and families rather than aggregates and the total community (Laffrey & Craig, 1995). In their survey of community health nursing research, Chalmers and Gregory (1995) found that most of the studies focused on individuals and aggregates and only a few on the community, that is, on "community mobilization, community development, community-wide health promotion, or policy development" (p. 607).

■ Community Health Nursing Research

An example of nursing research designed to promote health and prevent illness is Day's study to develop and evaluate a program to teach handicapped grade-one children about hand-washing in the prevention and control of contagious disease, such as colds, flu, and ear infections. Children in the study were taught when and how to wash their hands. Hand-washing skills were evaluated at 1, 3, and 6 months after teaching and were found to improve. The children had fewer visits to the doctor, took fewer prescribed medications, and had fewer illnesses than in the same period during the previous year. An interesting result of the study was that the children challenged the nurses about their hand-washing techniques with comments such as: "You can't touch me. I saw you blow your nose. Go wash your hands first" (AFNR Annual Report, 1989-1990).

Chalmers and Gregory (1995) conducted a literature review of community health nursing research from 1989 through 1993 and identified more than 400 references of which 238 were selected for further scrutiny as all contained an abstract, were in English, and were published studies. Of the 238 references, 29 studies were selected for content analysis based on meeting "the additional criterion of research conducted by Canadian nurse researchers as primary or co-investigators" (p. 602). The findings of some of the studies resulted in changes in practice; others had implications for change. In their survey of hospitals and community health units in Alberta, Field and Houston (1991) identified weaknesses in postpartum procedures and practices including changes in community health nursing practice to meet the information needs of new mothers. Poulin, Gyorkos, MacPhee, Cann and Bickerton (1992) designed and tested an interview schedule technique found to be successful in contact-tracing among injection drug users at risk for hepatitis B in rural areas. In their study of maternal stress related to repeated hospitalizations of physically disabled children, Ogden Burke, Costello, and Handley-Derry (1989) found implications for enhanced support of these families by community health nurses. An actual change in policy resulted from a study of discharge planning for postpartum mothers with referrals now being made to public health nurses by hospital maternity nurses and using public health liaison nurses as consultants as needed (Mitchell, Van Berkel, Adam, Ciliska, Sheppard, Baumann, Underwood, Walter, Gafni, Edwards & Southwell, 1993).

In her study of social support experienced by women caring for a cognitively impaired person, age 60 or older, Neufeld identified several barriers to asking for help. These included fear of refusal, fear of exposing a "family secret", and concern for reciprocity or how the caregiver would find time and energy to return the help. All of the caregivers said it was much better if people volunteered to help. Some stated they would never have asked for help and would never have made it through the caregiving if help had not been offered. With the increasing aging population in Canada, cutbacks in health care funding, and the trend to increase community care by family members, community health nurses need to be aware of such findings and consider the risk of overloading family caregivers and threatening their health. Neufeld points out that: "This would result in a greater demand on them and the system than would have been necessary had we initially helped them access sources of support and provided them with strong community support services for their caregiver role" (University of Alberta Faculty of Nursing Research and Scholarly Activities Report, 1993, p. 7).

Ross Kerr and Warren (1993) conducted a 3-year evaluation of 14 day-care programs for the elderly for Alberta health. Standardized instruments were used to interview 100 clients and 100 caregivers with 5 interviews each from the time of being on the waiting list to 6 months after admission to one of the 14 programs. Clients were tested for physical and cognitive function, quality of life and life satisfaction, perception of health and social support. Caregivers were tested for health status and burden; both caregivers and clients were tested for satisfaction with the program and their views on institutionalization. Satisfaction with the program was extremely high for both clients and caregivers. Caregivers mentioned the positive effects of the social, mental and physical stimulation on their family members and the critical effects of the respite for themselves. From preliminary analysis of the data, Ross Kerr stated:

> I don't believe adult day-care programs are an unnecessary frill, as some people have suggested. These programs provide much needed support to clients and caregivers who face daunting problems. I suspect that, without their desire to maintain community living and without these programs, many clients would have been institutionalized, though we really don't have evidence for that yet (University of Alberta Faculty of Nursing Research and Scholarly Activities Report, 1993, p. 14).

Based on her evaluation of an adult day-care program administered by the Victorian Order of Nurses (VON) for clients too disabled to qualify for other day-care programs, Strang found that respite care serves as a coping mechanism, not as a solution, for these highly stressed families. It provides a bridging function in moving the deteriorating, frail elderly from the community to an institution. She points out that if we can help to decrease the tremendous guilt involved in this transition, "we have made a major contribution to healthy-functioning families" (University of Alberta Faculty of Nursing Research and Scholarly Activities Report, 1993, p. 14).

Strang also evaluated foot care clinics administered by the VON with sponsoring organizations in the community, with the goal of maintaining mobility in the elderly. The findings demonstrated high client satisfaction with praise for the accessibility of the clinics and for their informal atmosphere and opportunity for socialization, as well as their effectiveness in enhancing mobility and health (University of Alberta Faculty of Nursing Research and Scholarly Activities Report, 1993).

Research-based practice has become even more important with diminishing health-care funds. The nursing profession must demonstrate how nursing interventions make a difference in improving the health status and health potential of individuals, families, groups, aggregates and communities. The only way this can be accomplished is through research followed by the dissemination of findings that are applied in practice. The nursing profession must move much more rapidly than in the past to research-based practice, which is a challenge with decreased funding for both health care and research. What has deterred nursing from increasing its research base? What can nurses do to promote and facilitate research-based practice?

■ Deterrents to Research-Based Nursing Practice

One of the major deterrents to research-based nursing practice has been the limited number of nurses prepared to conduct research. Although the number of nurses prepared at master's and doctoral levels has increased considerably in the past 15 years in Canada and the United States, the proportion of those nurses actually conducting research to strengthen the scientific base of practice is still limited. The number of nurses holding an earned doctorate in Canada increased from 81 in 1980 to 124 in 1982, to 193, in 1986, and to 247 in 1989; and the number of nurses involved in doctoral study increased from 72 in 1980 to 121 in 1982, to 224 in 1986, and to 265 in 1989 (Stinson, Larsen & MacPhail, 1984; Stinson, MacPhail & Larsen, 1988; Lamb & Stinson, 1990). Thus, the number of nurses with an earned doctorate increased by 53% from 1980 to 1982, by 56% from 1982 to 1986, and by 33% from 1986 to 1989; and the number of nurses engaged in doctoral study increased by 68% from 1980 to 1982, by 85% from 1982 to 1986, and by 18% from 1986 to 1989. The reasons for recent decreases in both categories are not known, but may be related to insufficient funding for graduate study and the lack of nursing doctoral programs in Canada until 1991. The establishment of five doctoral programs in nursing (University of Alberta, January 1991; University of British Columbia, September 1991; University of Toronto, September 1993; a joint program by McGill University and l'Université de Montréal, September 1993; and McMaster University, September 1994) should help to increase the number of Canadian nurses pursuing doctoral education. Also needed are more funds for doctoral study which is problematic with the cutbacks in funding for both health care and education in the provinces.

A second deterrent to conducting research in practice is difficulty in asking the research question, which is the most complex and the most important task of any researcher. Although research can solve problems, not all problems are research questions. The question, "Why don't staff nurses use the medication cart as it was designed?" reflects a problem. It may imply the question of how to get them to do it. The problem may be a management or morale problem, but as stated, it is not a research problem (Ellis, 1974). Two major types of questions are not researchable. These are value or "should" questions and "yes" or "no" questions. Types of researchable questions as identified by Wilson (1985, p. 117) are:

1. Why are things this way? For example, why do cancer patients without hope participate in painful experiments?

2. What would happen if? For example, what would happen if sex education were taught in all schools?
3. Which approach would work better? For example, is group or individual counselling more effective with clients who abuse alcohol?
4. Who might benefit from this? For example, would hospitalized children have faster recovery if parents were permitted and taught to participate in their care?

Dickoff, James and Wiedenbach (1986, p. 420) developed another categorization of types of research questions:

1. Factor-isolating or "naming". For example, what are the stages of the grieving process?
2. Factor-relating or "what is happening here?" For example, what is the relationship of parents' own childhood experiences to engaging in subsequent child abuse or neglect?
3. Situation-relating or "what will happen?" For example, will feedback training decrease suffering among chronic pain patients?
4. Situation-producing or "how can I make it happen?" For example, how can I intervene to prevent post-operative vomiting?

Brink and Wood (1983) define a researchable question as one that yields problem-solving information, produces new research, adds to theory, or improves practice. Lindeman and Schantz (1982) define it more narrowly as a question that can be answered by collecting observable data, that includes reference to the relationship between two or more variables, and that emanates from what is known about a phenomenon.

Defining researchable questions requires time and thought and a thorough search of the literature to determine what is known about the phenomenon being considered. Only in this way can one decide whether a question is worth investigating. Other factors that affect the feasibility of studying the question are time, availability of subjects, cooperation of others, facilities and equipment, money, research experience, and ethical considerations.

Many authors have identified insufficient time as an impediment to conducting research. It is a concern of faculty members who devote much time to teaching, curriculum development, committee work, and professional activities. It is also a concern of nursing staff in health care agencies who wish to participate in research (Alcock, Carroll & Goodman, 1990). Time for research may be limited by the orientation in nursing to "doing" and "being busy" and a tendency to want immediate results. Several writers have reported that nurses tend to want immediate results and fast action and have difficulty understanding that a hunch may not be borne out by research. On the other hand, educators may have difficulty using their time for research when they are accustomed to devoting it to teaching, curriculum study and revision, and committee work. This might be related to lagging commitment to research, as termed by Werley (1972).

Another deterrent to research in practice may be lack of access to clients. Access may be limited by physicians who have certain prerogatives in relation to their patients, whether hospitalized, in clinics or in offices. Access may also be limited by nurses who do not support or understand nursing research; nurses are in key positions to influence physicians, other nurses, administrators, and patients by educating them about the importance of research in nursing practice. This is not to suggest that clients' rights should not be protected, or that research proposals should not be subject to rigorous review for ethics and quality. Rather, it is to urge nurses to think about their influence on access to clients and the promotion of nursing research.

Insufficient funds to support research is an obstacle for all types of nursing research. It is a major problem in Canada because separate funding for nursing research has never been provided on the federal level, as in the United States where it has helped researchers gain experience in research design and grant writing needed to be able to compete in the larger arena (Gortner, 1986). On the federal level the Canadian government provides research funds for the social sciences and humanities, for the natural sciences and engineering, and for medicine and other health-related disciplines. Medical Research Council (MRC) funds are supposed to be available to health sciences other than medicine; however, most have been awarded to medicine. After vigorous lobbying by the Canadian Nurses Association (CNA) and the Canadian Association of University Schools of Nursing (CAUSN) for a number of years for representation on the MRC, nursing finally succeeded in having a nurse appointed in 1986. Despite success in obtaining some modifications in funding priorities for nursing research, a very limited proportion of MRC funding has been awarded to nurse investigators to date. The National Health Research and Development Program (NHRDP)-MRC Joint Program was developed a number of years ago to assist the profession in developing nursing research in university faculties of nursing. In the past 7 years the positions of 6 nursing scientists in several universities have been funded to allow them to conduct research. Recently in the final competition in this Joint Program, the positions of 6 nursing scientists in 3 universities (University of Alberta, l'Université de Montréal, and University of Toronto) were funded to allow them to conduct their own research and to assist nursing colleagues in undertaking research as well. One of the scientists at the University of Alberta also received an operating grant to support her research project, the first such grant to be awarded under the program.

Other research funding available to nurses is limited. Since 1985 the Canadian Nurses' Foundation (CNF) has offered small research grants, initially $1,500 and increased to a maximum of $5,000 in 1993. Two special grant categories were established with special funding in 1990, one for $15,000 in primary health care research and the other for $10,000 for pharmaceutical-related research. Through funding efforts of the CNF, 2 more $15,000 research grants became available in 1994 for research in any area of nursing practice. Although the grants available from the CNF still are relatively small, there is evidence of progress in the number of grant proposals received and the total amount of funds awarded annually: $9,602 in 1989; $21,582 in 1990; $37,500 in 1991; $75,823 in 1992; $51,221 in 1993; and $74,919 in 1994. The number of grant applications received increased from 23 in 1990 to 33 in 1992, decreased to 20 in 1993 and increased to 35 in 1994; and the number of grants awarded increased from 7 in 1990 to 15 in 1992, with a decrease to 10 in 1993 and an increase to 13 in 1994 (CNF Annual Reports, 1990, 1992, 1994). Fifty grant applications have been received in 1995, a 45% increase over 1994; awards are to be announced in December (Personal communication from Beverly Campbell, Executive Director, CNF, September 13, 1995).

Research funds may also be available through provincial nursing associations, but the amount tends to be even smaller. A few nursing researchers have been awarded "Career Scientist" grants by the Ontario Ministry of Health and the Research Division of the British Columbia Children's Hospital, which requires that the recipients devote 75% of their time to research and other scholarly activities. The latter requirement is a positive influence as it ensures that the investigator's research time is protected. Small grants may also be available from community health units, the Victorian Order of Nurses, hospital foundations, and endowment or other funds at the discretion of universities, hospitals and health units. Nurses may also apply for research funding through disease-oriented specialty organizations such as heart, lung, diabetes and cancer organizations, but they are competing with medicine and other health disciplines.

Another source of research funding for nursing became available in 1982 when the Alberta Foundation for Nursing Research (AFNR) was established by ministerial order as a response to lobbying by the Alberta Association of Registered Nurses (AARN) and nursing leaders of the University of Alberta and the University of Calgary. A fund of $1 million was allocated for use over a 5-year period, and a board of directors was appointed to establish research categories, guidelines and a review process, and to award and administer the funds. Support services to administer the fund were provided by the Alberta Department of Advanced Education. At the end of the 5 years, negotiations and political pressure succeeded in obtaining another $1 million for a 5-year period (to 1993). The first awards were made in the 1983-1984 fiscal year, and a total of $2,163,806 was awarded to Alberta nurses by the end of the 1991-1992 fiscal year. The amounts awarded per year and the number of awards made reflect remarkable progress, as shown by the allocation of $19,015 to 7 recipients in the first year (1983-1984); $280,404 for 33 awards in 1988-1989; $392,675 for 29 awards in 1990-1991; and $314,499 for 26 awards in 1991-1992 (Alberta

Foundation for Nursing Research, 1990-1991 and 1991-1992). In some grant categories, the amounts available were increased as new ideas evolved and experience showed that original amounts were insufficient to achieve the research objectives. For example, the maximum award for the Research Project category was increased from $25,000 to $50,000 and then to $85,000; and the maximum duration was increased from 2 to 3 years in the 1989-1990 fiscal year (AFNR, 1989-1990).

In addition to having a significant effect on the development of nursing research in Alberta, the AFNR has helped to increase the visibility of Alberta nursing researchers because a significant number of AFNR-funded studies have been published and presented at national and international research conferences. With the establishment of AFNR, Alberta became the first and only province or state worldwide to designate funds exclusively for nursing research. This is also the first research funding endeavour in Canada in which nurses have had a primary role in reviewing grant proposals and awarding funds. Sadly, with recent cutbacks in funding for research, education and health care by the Alberta Legislature, the future of the AFNR is tenuous as originally structured. Nurses in Alberta are working toward the development of a new structure which would continue to support funding for nursing research. This structure is seen as amalgamating the efforts of the AARN, the Alberta Nurses Educational Trust and the present arrangements for the AFNR. It remains to be seen how this initiative will develop in the future.

A final deterrent to achieving the goal of research-based practice pertains to the utilization of research findings in practice settings. Because such a limited proportion of nurses are prepared to conduct research and interpret research findings, there is need for intermediary mechanisms to assist nursing staff in interpreting and applying research findings in practice. There is also need for changes in values and incentives within health-care agencies to recognize and reward research-based nursing practice. Alcock, Carroll and Goodman (1990) conducted a study of staff nurses in Ontario to determine their perceptions of: the value of nursing research, their role in nursing research, their interest in nursing research, their research experience, and the research climate in their employing agency. Using a pretested questionnaire and a calculated proportionate sample, the survey was directed to 4 groups of staff nurses: public health nurses; home care/visiting nurses; nurses in teaching hospitals; and nurses in non-teaching hospitals. Although the return rate of 45% was low, differences were found among the groups with a 63% return from public health nurses; 53% by home care/visiting nurses; 47% by non-teaching hospital nurses; and 39% by teaching hospital nurses. Nurses prepared at the baccalaureate level placed more value on nursing research than those prepared at the diploma and certificate levels, and public health nurses perceived the value significantly higher than nurses in hospitals. Although 93% of the respondents perceived they have a role in applying research findings in practice, most were not informed about the research milieu in their agencies, about one-third did not read research literature, and most perceived lack of a supportive research climate in their agencies. Under such circumstances, implementation of research-based changes in practice is likely to be limited.

There is need for changes in values and incentives within health-care agencies to recognize and reward research and research-based practice. Nursing administrators play a key role in creating a supportive research climate. McClure (1981) has noted that to support research a nurse executive requires a substantial knowledge of research methods and research literature, not only to provide a climate that supports research, but also to make the arrangements necessary for studies to proceed. She believes that commitment of time and energy by the nurse executive is essential to promoting and facilitating research and the application of research findings in practice. With the cutbacks in funding for health care and research, low priority may be given to research and research-based practice in budget planning, but "the cost effectiveness of implementing changes, based on research findings that contribute to improved outcomes, must be taken into consideration" (Alcock, Carroll, & Goodman, 1990, p. 15).

■ Strategies to Promote Research and Research-Based Practice

The deterrents identified in relation to the development of research and the promotion of research-based practice in themselves suggest possible solutions. Implementation of solutions or strategies will require strong commitment and determination by all nurses, not just nurses involved in research or who want to conduct research.

A basic requirement is to increase the proportion of nurses who appreciate the importance of research, understand research methods, and have beginning ability to evaluate research reports critically. This implies a need for more baccalaureate-prepared nurses, which is consistent with the nursing profession's goal for entry to practice by the year 2000. Remarkable progress has been made within the past 3 years particularly, in developing collaborative programs between university faculties/schools of nursing and diploma programs in the western provinces and the Atlantic region provinces, designed to increase, greatly, opportunities for baccalaureate education in nursing.

A second strategy is to increase the proportion of nurses prepared at the master's and doctoral levels. More funding is needed to increase enrollments, for which all nurses should lobby. Some nursing faculty members have competed successfully for funds to support research training and research projects; however, the number has been small and the proportion almost infinitesimal when compared with funding for medicine and other disciplines. In addition to increasing enrollments, attention must be given to the quality of the research preparation within graduate programs, to providing resources for faculty to increase research competence and grantsmanship skills, and to holding faculty members accountable for conducting research and disseminating their findings.

The Canadian Nurses Association (CNA) has been a strong proponent of nursing research, particularly since the 1960s. The CNA Board of Directors allocated $10,000 to support the establishment of the Canadian Nurses' Foundation (CNF) in 1962 to serve as a mechanism to receive funds and award them on a competitive basis to nurses admitted to baccalaureate and graduate programs. Funds are raised through membership dues and appeals for donations from individuals, associations and corporations. In 1984 the CNF added a small research grants program to which reference was made previously. Although the funds available do not meet the needs, the CNF plays an important role in encouraging nurses to pursue baccalaureate and graduate education and to undertake small research projects and develop grant-writing skills. Other examples of the CNA's support of nursing research are (1) establishment of a nursing research committee in 1971 that became a standing committee in 1978; (2) amendment of CNA bylaws in 1976 to include a member-at-large for nursing research on the board of directors; (3) publication of the first inventory of Canadian nursing doctoral statistics in 1980 with updates in 1982, 1986 and 1989; (4) publication of CNA's *Research Imperative for Nursing in Canada*, a strategic plan for the development of nursing research prepared by the Research Committee and approved by the board of directors in 1984 and revised in 1990; and (5) vigorous lobbying over the years for recognition and funding of nursing research and graduate education to prepare more nurses to conduct research.

Many strategies to create a research climate in practice settings, and to promote research-based practice, have been effective. One is the appointment of a clinical nurse researcher who works with the nursing staff to formulate research questions, who designs and conducts research projects, and who involves staff members in the process. The role includes educating staff members about nursing research and its importance and potential for improving practice, and establishing a proper research-review process for screening nursing research proposals before they are sent on to the agency review committee. The role also includes interpreting nursing research to other disciplines, notably medicine; serving on the agency's research review committee; ensuring that the research-review process is rigorous; and assisting in the application of valid and reliable research findings. The enactment of such a role requires a nurse prepared at the doctoral level who is not only competent in designing and conducting research, but also skilled in communication and in effecting planned change. It also requires strong administrative support, ability to create a research climate that encourages questioning current practices, readiness to test different nursing approaches, and nursing staff interested in trying new approaches. Clarke (1995) points out that this role is not yet prevalent in community health nursing agencies, but may be assumed by a nursing research director or a clinical nurse specialist in some agencies or a nursing researcher may be engaged as a consultant on a part-time or contractual basis. Another approach is a researcher in a joint appointment with the cost shared by the community health agency and a university faculty/school of nursing. This approach has been applied effectively by a number of universities (Alberta, British Columbia, Calgary, Dalhousie, Manitoba, McGill, McMaster, Ottawa and Toronto) in collaboration with both community health agencies and hospitals.

The provision of research consultation is a strategy found to be effective in promoting quality research and research-based practice. Also important are library resources, educationally prepared nurses, funding, and time to be involved in research endeavours (Thurston, Tenove & Church, 1990; Fitch, 1992; Rosswurm, 1992; Clarke, 1995). Research consultation has been provided to Saskatchewan nurses through the Saskatchewan Nursing Research Unit, established in 1983 with joint sponsorship by the University of Saskatchewan College of Nursing, the Saskatchewan Registered Nurses Association, and the Saskatchewan Union of Nurses. Similar services have been provided by the Manitoba Nursing Research Unit, funded jointly by the University of Manitoba School of Nursing and the Manitoba Association of Registered Nurses, beginning in 1985; and to nurses in all parts of Alberta for 1 year (1986-1987) through a special grant that supported a nursing research consultant and was administered through the Alberta Foundation for Nursing Research (AFNR). The idea emanated from the AFNR board of directors who were concerned that nurses in many health care agencies lacked consultation resources. Dr. Mary Houston, who then held an appointment in the University of Lethbridge School of Nursing, served as the consultant on a full-time basis. All of these programs demonstrated the need for this type of service to increase and enhance research. In the first 6 months of the Alberta project, research consultation was provided to more than 100 nurses; 35% were from health care agencies, 26% from colleges and universities, and 12% from professional associations and committees (AFNR, 1987). The response was gratifying and reflected a great need which still exists, as identified by the AFNR board of directors who requested the Alberta Association of Registered Nurses (AARN) "to explore the possibility of creating a Nursing Research Consultant position" (AFNR Annual Report, 1990-1991, p. 2). Such a position was established by the Registered Nurses Association of British Columbia in 1988 and Dr. Heather Clarke has demonstrated clearly the potentialities and feasibility of the role in that province. Fiscal constraints have precluded its development in Alberta to date where universities continue to provide some consultation through joint appointees and other collaborative arrangements; however, this does not meet all of the identified needs in that province.

Pepler (1992) describes a strategy used in a major teaching hospital to promote research-based practice. As a consultant in nursing research in that setting, she developed a 24-hour educational program presented over a 12-week period that is available to nursing staff from other hospitals in Montreal as well as to the Royal Victoria Hospital staff. It has "helped nurses gain the knowledge and skills to find, interpret and judge research findings and to change their world of practice" (Pepler, 1992, p. 27). Other outcomes reported are greater use of research consultation services, ability to understand research presentations at conferences, and increased support for nursing research and research-based practice. Such a program could be made available to nursing staff in community health and other health care agencies.

A strategy emphasized by Clarke (1995) for promoting research and research-based practice is a research committee within a health care agency. Such a committee may promote or provide research-based education for nursing staff; present research findings; publish a research newsletter; and provide consultation on research proposal writing; however, to fulfill such functions requires considerable research expertise. Other conditions considered to be vitally important within an agency are adequate release time and access to library resources, secretarial services and computers. A survey of 174 health care agencies in British Columbia, including 28 community health departments, found very limited development of such support services to promote and facilitate the development of nursing research programs and research-based practice. (RNABC, 1993).

Unit-based research roundtable discussions, undertaken jointly by faculty and unit leaders, are another approach to increase awareness of the relevance of research to practice and to disseminate research findings to nursing staff and nursing students (Janken, Dufault & Yeaw, 1988). Although the process required time, patience and persistence, they found it resulted in more favourable attitudes toward research, increased application of research findings in practice, improved communications, and the development of a new respect between staff and students.

A strategy tried by some nursing researchers is to provide an interpretation of research findings in language that nursing staff can understand. Kirchhoff (1983) favours this approach by providing short summaries of results in clinically-oriented journals; however, the summaries must be written by a competent researcher. The American Association of Critical Care Nurses has used this approach in their clinical journal, *Focus,* by including reviews of nursing studies with suggestions for practice. The *Western Journal of Nursing Research* used a similar strategy by publishing a column, "Using Research in Practice." Haller, Reynolds and Horsley (1979) used research-based protocols for nursing staff to follow in several Michigan hospitals as another approach to promoting research-based practice. It is essential to have a scholarly critique of the original research and ensure that nursing staff and students recognize that such protocols and suggestions for practice cannot be applied without the interim step of interpretation by a skilled researcher. Kirchhoff (1983) also suggests that research conferences include a response to a research report entitled "Clinical Application," presented by a skilled researcher-clinician. Such an approach might encourage more nursing staff members to attend research conferences.

Another strategy to stimulate the development of research and research-based practice is organizing research interest groups within the professional organization or within a health-care agency or group of agencies. They require leaders with research expertise to help the group define purposes. Is it to learn to read and apply research findings, to conduct research, or both? Should there be one general research group, or should there be smaller groups focused on particular interests? Experience with such interest groups has demonstrated great potential when leadership is provided by nurses knowledgeable about research methods and able to help the group identify researchable practice problems. Other approaches used in health-care agencies are organizing research rounds, holding research presentations over lunch hour, and forming journal clubs in which research discussion is led by a competent investigator. Another technique is to involve staff in data collection so they learn what is involved in research to some extent and that research results are not immediately forthcoming.

Staff participation in research review and ethical clearance can be a valuable learning opportunity if under the direction and guidance of a competent nursing researcher who works with the staff to help them understand all the factors that must be considered. One must assess the quality of a research proposal in order to give ethical clearance; if the study is not well designed it is not ethical to take clients' or subjects' time. This implies that the nursing researcher must select a committee and educate the members about the review process. They need basic knowledge of research and the requirements for reviewing and interpreting nursing research, which implies that members have at least a baccalaureate degree. Guidelines for research review have been developed in some health-care agencies, such as the University of Alberta Hospitals, where a clinical nurse researcher provides leadership in the process. These guidelines are available to nurses involved or interested in promoting and facilitating research in other agencies.

Researchers can share their findings through written media as well as verbal presentations. They can be published in a health care agency's monthly newsletter. Many nursing departments have a publication of some type in which a column can be devoted to research. Professional associations' newsletters have included such a column to reach more nurses. Both should be done under the guidance of a competent researcher to ensure that quality is maintained and that terminology is appropriate for neophytes in research.

In the process of learning about nursing research, the nursing staff and students become familiar with nursing research journals. These include *Nursing Research, Research in Nursing and Health, Advances in Nursing Science, Image: The Journal of Nursing Scholarship, Western Journal of Nursing Research,* and *Clinical Nursing Research.* All are published in the United States, but since 1987 the *Western Journal of Nursing Re-*

search has been edited at the University of Alberta by Pamela Brink and Marilynn Wood of the Faculty of Nursing. *Clinical Nursing Research* is a journal launched in 1992 to focus on clinical practice problems, encourage discussion among practitioners, identify potential clinical application of the latest scholarly research, and disseminate research findings of particular interest to practising nurses. It is edited at the University of Alberta by Marilynn Wood and Pat Hayes. The *Canadian Journal of Nursing Research* (formerly *Nursing Papers*) is the only Canadian nursing research journal. It has been edited and published through McGill University since 1968. Although its readership has been limited, it is increasing gradually with more doctorally prepared nurses conducting research and sharing their findings. Thus, opportunities are increasing to publish nursing research, promote and facilitate the application of valid and reliable findings in practice, and progress toward the goal of research-based nursing practice.

■ Future of Research-Based Nursing Practice

The progress made in increasing the number of nurses prepared to conduct research and the number and quality of practice-oriented studies undertaken by nursing researchers, is encouraging. Nonetheless, there is need for practising nurses, as individuals and as members of their professional organizations, to promote and support the advancement of nursing knowledge through research and the improvement of nursing practice and health care through application of valid and reliable research findings in practice. As we approach the 21st century with increasing competition for scarce financial resources, strong commitment to the goal will be required of all nurses—practitioners, educators, administrators and researchers—to continue to strengthen the research base of nursing practice.

■ References

Alberta Foundation for Nursing Research. (1986-1987). *Annual report.* Edmonton, Alberta: The Foundation.
Alberta Foundation for Nursing Research. (1989-1990). *Annual report.* Edmonton, Alberta: The Foundation.
Alberta Foundation for Nursing Research. (1990-1991). *Annual report.* Edmonton, Alberta: The Foundation.
Alberta Foundation for Nursing Research. (1991-1992). *Annual report.* Edmonton, Alberta: The Foundation.
Alcock, D., Carroll, G., & Goodman, M. (1990). Staff nurses' perceptions of factors influencing their role in research. *The Canadian Journal of Nursing Research, 22*(4), 7-18.
Brink, P.J., & Wood, M.J. (1983). *Basic steps in planning nursing research: From question to proposal* (2nd ed). Belmont, CA: Wadsworth Health Services.
Canadian Nurses' Foundation. (1990). *1990 annual report.* Ottawa, Ontario: The Foundation.
Canadian Nurses' Foundation. (1992). *1992 annual report.* Ottawa, Ontario: The Foundation.
Chalmers, K.I., & Gregory, D.M. (1995). Community health nursing research: Theoretical and practical challenges. In M.J. Stewart (Ed.), *Community nursing: Promoting Canadians' health* (pp. 600-617). Toronto: W.B. Saunders Canada.

Clarke, H.F. (1995). Research-based practice in community health nursing. In M.J. Stewart (Ed.), *Community nursing: Promoting Canadians' health* (pp. 577-599). Toronto: W.B. Saunders Canada.

Dickoff, J., James, P., & Wiedenbach, E. (1968). Theory in a practice discipline: Part 1. Practice-oriented theory. *Nursing Research, 17*(5), 415-435.

Ellis, R. (1974). Asking the research question. In: *Issues in research: Social, professional and methodological* (pp. 31-35). Kansas City, MO: American Nurses Association.

Field, P.A., & Houston, M. (1991). Teaching and support: Nursing input in the postpartum period. *International Journal of Nursing Studies, 28*(2), 131-144.

Fitch, M. (1992). Five years in the life of a nursing research and professional development division. *Canadian Journal of Nursing Administration, 5*(2), 20-26.

Gortner, S.R. (1986). Impact of the Division of Nursing on research development in the United States. In S.M. Stinson & J.C. Kerr (Eds.), *International issues in nursing research* (pp. 113-130). London: Croom Helm.

Haller, K.B., Reynolds, M.A., & Horsley, J.A. (1979). Developing research-based innovation protocols: Process, criteria and issues. *Research in Nursing and Health, 2*(2), 45-51.

Janken, J.K., Dufault, M.A., & Yeaw, E.M. (1988). Research round tables: Increasing student/staff awareness of the relevancy of research to practice. *Journal of Professional Nursing, 4*(3), 186-191.

Kirchhoff, K.T. (1983). Using research in practice: Should staff nurses be expected to use research? *Western Journal of Nursing Research, 5*(3), 245-247.

Laffrey, S.C., & Craig, D.M. (1995). Health promotion for communities and aggregates: An integrated model. In M.J. Stewart (Ed.), *Community nursing: Promoting Canadians' health* (pp. 125-145). Toronto: W.B. Saunders Canada.

Lamb, M.A., & Stinson, S.M. (1990). *Canadian nursing doctoral statistics: 1989 update.* Ottawa, Ontario: Canadian Nurses Association.

Lindeman, C.A., & Schantz, D. (1982). The research question. *Journal of Nursing Administration, 12*(1), 6-10.

McClure, M.L. (1981). Promoting practice-based research: A critical need. *Journal of Nursing Administration, 11*(11 & 12), 66-70.

Mitchell, A., Van Berkel, C., Adam, V., Ciliska, D., Sheppard, K., Baumann, A., Underwood, J., Walter, S., Gafni, A., Edwards, N., & Southwell, D. (1993). Comparison of liaison and staff nurses in discharge referrals of postpartum patients for public health nursing follow-up. *Nursing Research, 42*(4), 245-249.

Ogden Burke, S., Costello, E., & Handley-Derry, M. (1989). Maternal stress and repeated hospitalizations of children who are physically disabled. *Children's Health Care, 18*(2), 82-90.

Pepler, C. (1992). Fostering change through education. *The Canadian Nurse, 88*(1), 25-27.

Poulin, C., Gyorkos, T., MacPhee, J., Cann, B., & Bickerton, J. (1992). Contact-tracing among injection drug users in a rural area. *Canadian Journal of Public Health, 83*(2), 106-108.

Registered Nurses Association of British Columbia (1993). *Nursing and research in clinical agencies: A B.C. survey.* Vancouver: The Association.

Rosswurm, M.A. (1992). A research-based practice model in a hospital setting. *Journal of Nursing Administration, 22*(3), 57-59.

Schlotfeldt, R.M. (1971). The significance of empirical research for nursing. *Nursing Research, 20*(2), 140-142.

Stinson, S.M., Larsen, J., & MacPhail, J. (1984). *Canadian nursing doctoral statistics: 1982 update.* Ottawa, Ontario: Canadian Nurses Association.

Stinson, S.M., MacPhail, J., & Larsen, J. (1988). *Canadian nursing doctoral statistics: 1986 update.* Ottawa, Ontario: Canadian Nurses Association.

Thurston, N., Tenove, S., & Church, J. (1990). Hospital nursing research is alive and flourishing. *Nursing Management, 21*(5), 50-54.

University of Alberta Faculty of Nursing Research and Scholarly Activities Report, Caring for the Elderly, 1993. Available from the Faculty of Nursing, University of Alberta, Clinical Sciences Building, Edmonton, Alberta, T6G 2G3.

Werley, H. (1972). This I believe about clinical nursing research. *Nursing Outlook, 20*(11), 718-722.

Wilson, H.S. (1985). *Research in nursing.* Don Mills, Ontario: Addison-Wesley Publishing Company.

7

CURRENT AND FUTURE CHALLENGES IN COMMUNITY HEALTH NURSING

JANET ROSS KERR AND JANNETTA MACPHAIL

In the modern context, community health nursing has been a recognized and viable field of practice for nurses since the formal organization of nursing as a profession in Canada. Following World War I, it was recognized that nurses were key professionals to implement strategies designed to protect the health of the public. The new value placed upon health resulted from the impact of the wartime death toll, concern at the large number of young men who were declared unhealthy and unfit for war service and the devastating consequences of the worldwide Spanish influenza epidemic between 1917 and 1919. The League of Red Cross Societies adopted a resolution making promotion of health and prevention of disease a major peacetime project. In Canada, grants to six universities by the Canadian Red Cross Society became the stimulus for the development of university level education in public health nursing for nurses. These specialized courses in public health nursing continued after the 3-year term of the Red Cross grants in 5 of the institutions, became part of an existing degree program in one institution and eventually led to degree programs in the other 4 institutions.

Before the registration of nurses, nurses were independent entrepreneurs who were privately engaged to care for people in their homes. The rise in the scope and sophistication of health care centred in the hospital over the past century has meant that community health nursing, both in terms of health promotion and disease prevention for the well and care in the home for the ill, was relegated to a back seat in the health care arena. The development of government responsibility for health care as reflected in federal legislation to establish a national health insurance program further entrenched a system of health care based on the primacy of acute care interventions for disease and the centrality of physicians' services. These characteristics were the outcome of the designation of hospital care and physicians' services for reimbursement under the passage of acts which laid the foundation for national health insurance; these acts took effect in 1957 for hospital care and in 1968 for medical care. As a result of the form of national health insurance legislation, an inordinate degree of control over the health system was wielded by physicians who would serve as gatekeepers to health care services. Nurses gained a prominent place in the hospital-based system, but because of the organization of health services imposed by the federal legislation, their roles were limited because they were not specifically identified for reimbursement and were therefore subject to the control of hospitals and indirectly of physicians.

The need for the health consumer to see a physician in order to receive reimbursable services left no room for the most effective and efficient use of health professionals. Nurses have argued for a considerable length of time for a stronger preventive and health promotion thrust in health care, as well as for more appropriate roles for nurses in the system. In the document *Putting Health into Health Care* by the Canadian Nurses Association (CNA), the CNA made a powerful case for better treatment of consumers and utilization of nurses. The passage of the Canada Health Act of 1984 allowed for reimbursement for the services of "health practitioners." This category could include both nurses and other health professionals such as physiotherapists. That the clause identifying that provinces could receive reimbursement for the services of "health practitioners" was included in the Act stands as a tribute to the work of the CNA. The CNA influenced the federal government to include this matter through the publication referred to above and through intensive lobbying efforts to secure passage of the "health practitioner" amendment. Because health is the constitutional responsibility of the provinces, federal health statutes take the form of enabling legislation to allow provinces to receive federal funds to support health care under conditions laid down by the national government. Thus, in order for the health practitioner clause to be implemented, a province would need to decide to implement it. After more than a decade following the legislation, no province has yet implemented this section of the legislation.

The health care reform movement which is currently sweeping the country has been largely driven by the need to eliminate deficit financing and ultimately accumulated provincial debt loads. At the federal level, funding provided to the provinces has also been markedly reduced for similar reasons. Although the national program of health insurance remains a highly popular initiative of the federal and provincial governments, and polls have shown that citizens are concerned by what is perceived to be excessive slashing of health programs and services, government 'belt-tightening' appears to have hit a popular chord in most areas. This seeming contradiction may have resulted from years of excess and inefficiency, both within government circles and within the health system. As a result of tightening the reins of health budgets in the belief that substantial cost savings can be realized in a restructured system, commitment has emerged in some provinces to move the primary locus of health care from hospital to community settings with greater emphasis upon home care.

The process of restructuring the health system is exceedingly complex. In Alberta, major restructuring and cost-cutting efforts have surpassed those of any other province to date. Initiated in 1993 and extending over a four-year period, the effects of the 20% reduction in health care costs have been striking. From the outset, the downsizing has led to the loss of thousands of professional and nonprofessional jobs. Most notable among professional job losses have been those of the nurses employed in the acute health care sector in hospitals. The province of Ontario is now embarking upon a similar budget reduction process in all of its social institutions and other provinces have been engaged in restructuring, such as in Saskatchewan where the health system has been regionalized and in Quebec, New Brunswick, and Newfoundland where major downsizing efforts have been announced. It is likely that the constraints under which the health system has operated for almost four decades since the implementation of national health insurance have been responsible, at least in part, for the significant increases in costs over time. These constraints relate primarily to a number of factors. First, great expenditures are incurred when consumers are required by the system to see a physician to gain access to health care, when an alternative, lower cost and in many cases, more appropriate health professional could be consulted. Just as the use of other health professionals needs to be appropriate, the use of physicians in a health system truly rationalized for effective and efficient operation also needs to make the best use of the professional skill and expertise of generalist and specialist physicians. Second, the direction of an inordinately high proportion of funds expended for health care to acute care and treatment with very little to prevention and health promotion has represented another important historical constraint upon the system. Finally, the entrenchment of a fee-for-service system for physicians through the provisions of the provincial health insurance plans and the federal legislation meant that physicians would be remunerated on a task centred basis rather than on a more person-centred basis. That this was a very expensive method of remunerating physicians for their services became apparent over time, as physician costs were an important component of the rise in the cost of health services in the contemporary context. The establishment of fee-for-service remuneration for physicians through legislation has also had a stifling effect on changes in the way in which other health professionals could practise and on the operation of the health care system in general.

■ The Changing Focus of Professional Nursing Practice

While for many years most nurses have been employed in hospitals with a much smaller percentage in the community health sector, it seems clear that major changes in employment patterns in the nursing workforce are about to occur. In provinces which are at the forefront of health care reform, large numbers of nurses have lost their positions in hospitals as a consequence of significant reductions in the capacity of those institutions. At the same time those with an appropriate background of education and experience are finding employment in the community, primarily in the home care sector. Just what the approaches will be to using nurses to their full capacity are still unclear. However, some initiatives to employ highly qualified nurses more effectively in the health system are being seen. In Alberta, Bill 5, the Public Health Amendment Act was passed in 1995. This Act has passed third reading and plans are to proclaim it at the same time as the regulations are approved. This Act will allow registered nurses to provide extended health services in designated employment settings in accordance with regulations. Extended services refer to diagnosis, treatment of common health problems, drug therapy, emergency services and referral. However, the Alberta Medical Association has mounted vociferous opposition to the legislation, indicating that it is not in the public interest. One section of concern is one referring to liability, which will likely be amended before the act receives Royal Assent and is proclaimed. Of further interest, the Alberta Minister of Health has indicated to the President of the Alberta Association of Registered Nurses not only that she will continue to support the legislation and intends to see it proclaimed, but also that she supports the employment of registered nurses in extended practice if a need for their services is identified by the health regions in the province regardless of geographic location (Personal communication, Dr. Lillian Douglass, December 4, 1995). Although the latter change would likely occur at a later date, it seems reasonable to envision the extension of this Act to urban areas and other parts of the province with reorganization and rationalization of all medical and health services.

Physicians are influential, well-organized, and lobby governments very effectively in areas of concern to them. In the past, they have opposed efforts to include services provided by nurses as being among those eligible for direct reimbursement in provincial health-care plans. Therefore it will not be easy for provincial governments, even those which intend to change existing services in the best possible way, to strike a balance between the interests of physicians who are highly respected and who wield considerable power in the community with the interests of other parties. These include those of other health professionals including nurses who have been relegated to roles that in many cases do not allow them to use their knowledge and skills to the maximum benefit of the health-care consumer. Developing the most effective and efficient health system at the least possible cost is important. Nurses provide a viable and cost-effective alternative in delivering many health-care services, particularly those involving health promotion, health maintenance and counselling activities relative to health. Health-care legislation has imposed financial constraints on nursing roles and functions over a lengthy period of time. This has meant that change that might have occurred naturally in a free and open health-care environment has not occurred. To date, powerful physician-dominated lobby groups have prevented major departures from the physician-centred health system maintained through the force of health insurance financing legislation. Nurses have also demonstrated their effectiveness at lobbying and are finding that politicians are increasingly interested in the point of view of the nursing profession. It is critical that politicians understand the actual and potential contributions of nurses to the health system. Since other alternative health providers in a number of specialized areas could provide effective and efficient services to benefit the consumer and the system as a whole, politicians need to understand the scope of what these various groups have to offer as well as to develop the political will to restructure the system so that their services are factored into a system that operates smoothly and responsibly. Governments will be forced to consider alternatives, despite the pressure to resist change, as the limits of the public purse and the demand for improved health are recognized.

The worldwide movement to implement primary health care initiated by the World Health Organization (1978) envisioned primary health care as

> essential health care based on practical, scientifically sound and socially acceptable methods and technology made universally accessible to individuals and families in the community through their full participation and at a cost that the community and country can afford to maintain at every stage of their development in the spirit of self-reliance and self-determination (p. 21).

Community health nurses have been seen as critical to the implementation of primary health care in Canada and elsewhere, as articulated by Dr. Hafdan Mahler, Director-General of WHO (1985). The CNA (1988) identified fundamental principles of PHC as health promotion, public participation, intersectoral and interdisciplinary collaboration, accessibility and appropriate technology. Even though health reform has been driven by right wing efforts to reduce health spending and eliminate deficit financing, as the process unfolds it is clear that its philosophical orientation is based upon the principles of primary health care. The shift to the community has been accompanied by goals that have been variously expressed as developing a seamless health system, increasing public participation in health policy development as well as in the process of care, focusing upon health promotion and developing more effective partnerships between the health professions and other groups interested in health at all levels. Although some of these goals raise issues of concern for the established health professions including nursing, the nursing profession to its credit has supported initiatives in all five areas of the PHC principles. In terms of interdisciplinary collaboration, there are clearly tensions in the move to a primary health care model with relationships between medicine and nursing. Physicians are anxious about the proposed changes and there is a perception on their part that they stand to lose ground financially if they relinquish the control they have held under the current system. They fear that if they approve new forms of remuneration for their services, they would become powerless health system employees rather than independent entrepreneurs exercising considerable control as they bill the system for their services. Nurses are clearly looking forward to more collaborative working relationships with physicians and those in other health disciplines as the system is rationalized and reorganized with a view to improved outcomes for the health consumer. Clearly, multidisciplinary team building will be important in moving to collaborative community health practice.

Community health nursing practice is likely to undergo tremendous change in the months and years to come in all regions of the country. The organized profession is in the forefront of this change, and Stewart (1995) has identified some excellent examples of the kinds of projects which the professional associations have undertaken to explore and promote application of the principles of primary health care in community health nursing practice. The health needs assessment being carried out in the Cheticamp Primary Health Care Project has involved a number of strategies to involve people in putting forward their needs, including surveys, focus groups, community forum and kitchen table discussions (Stewart, 1995). Although there was little movement in the provinces to implement the "health practitioner" clause in the Canada Health Act of 1984, the above-noted development of legislation to amend the Public Health Act in Alberta to allow nurses to practise in advanced roles is encouraging. It is important to develop new approaches to delivering health care. The swing of the pendulum back to the home from the hospital will require structural changes in the organization of the system, in the modes of care, and in the ways in which providers are asked to collaborate to provide the most effective services possible for the health consumer.

■ Education for Community Health Nursing Practice

The history of nursing education has been characterized by the search for appropriate standards to improve the quality of nursing education programs. Community health nursing was the stimulus for the movement of nursing education into the universities in 1919 and over time was a potent force in the development of degree programs in nursing in every province. Support for the entry to practice position of the profession, which specified that all new graduates should be prepared for nursing practice in university-level programs by the year 2000, was also driven by the need to develop a stronger focus in community health nursing in nursing programs. Given that professional practice is rapidly moving to support a much higher proportion of nurses working in the community that in the past, the supportive educational component at the university level is imperative. The remarkable progress made since 1991 in moving toward the entry to practice goal through collaboration between university and diploma nursing programs will undoubtedly continue as there is a groundswell of activity in this area nationally. The primary goal of this major change in nursing education programs is the development of an effective system of primary health care as we move toward the 21st century. The nursing profession has been in the forefront of the entry to practice and PHC movements and recognizes the relationship between the need for education to support nurses practising in a system in which the PHC approach is central. There are many challenges that require careful thought and concerted action by politically astute leaders and members of the profession.

The preparation of nurses as clinical specialists who can serve as expert practitioners and teachers has been a critical need for some time. In Ontario, special programs for the development of nurse practitioners at the post-baccalaureate level are underway. The achievement of the entry to practice position is conditioned to a certain extent by the accessibility and availability of graduate work in nursing. Therefore, graduate programs strong in clinical and research preparation are key elements in expanding and strengthening the ranks of well-prepared clinical nurse specialists in health organizations and agencies. The development and expansion of university programs in nursing at the baccalaureate level cannot be accomplished without the infusion of considerable numbers of faculty prepared at the master's and doctoral levels. Thus, the development of graduate programs must go hand in hand with the new developments in undergraduate degree programs.

Master's programs have been established on a regional basis across the country and offer opportunities for advanced preparation in community health nursing. A primary issue in the 35 years since the first master's degree program in nursing was established at the University of Western Ontario has been program capacity and geographic accessibility of programs. With the availability and growing affordability of interactive videoconference technology, the demand for distance delivery of masters' programs in nursing confirms the need for greater availability of this level of education in nursing across a wider geographic area. The development of a strong clinical base in masters' degree programs was slow to develop initially, since the early programs offered only functional specialization in nursing education and nursing administration. Clinical concentration in areas of interest including community health nursing has become an important goal in programs and virtually all seek to prepare graduates for an advanced level of nursing practice.

The establishment of 5 doctoral programs in nursing in Canada since the first program was established at the University of Alberta in 1991 was a development that was long overdue. There have been some increases in research funds and productivity in university schools and faculties of nursing involved in developing graduate programs over the past 2 decades. This has occurred gradually as a result of an increasing number of nurses with preparation in research and the wider availability of funding for nursing research investigations. The development of a strong research thrust in faculties of nursing is critical to the development of outstanding graduate programs in nursing, and to developing strength in clinical areas of practice.

The foregoing attests to the tremendous range of issues in nursing education. In the context of health care reform, there are exciting opportunities for the profession as restructuring of all services is occurring at a rapid rate. With the associated transition to a much greater proportion of health services being offered in the community, direct access to nursing services is likely to be permitted in at least some regions of the country. With fundamental changes in patterns of practice, nursing education at the baccalaureate, master's, and doctoral levels will need to be responsive to the necessity for change as well to prepare practitioners to function in advanced practice roles in the future. It is unlikely that there will be any reversal of the trend toward specialization in nursing. With continued development and incorporation of new knowledge into professional practice, it will be important to ensure that there is appropriate educational support for nurses in various specialties. In this climate of change, the opportunities for the profession in the future are limitless. It is likely that the strong leadership, which has always characterized the profession, will continue to facilitate the adaptation and development of systems of nursing education to prepare practitioners to meet the needs of health care consumers of the future.

Primary Health Care Concepts in the Basic Undergraduate Curriculum

A major challenge for the immediate future is integrating primary health care (PHC) concepts in the basic curriculum with concomitant changes in the practice opportunities provided students to enable them to implement the concepts. This will require collaboration by nursing educators with leaders in a much broader variety of community settings than the traditional community health agencies, as well as vision of the potentialities of PHC for changing health care delivery in Canada.

Edwards and Craig (1987) identified not only minimal integration of PHC concepts in the curricula of university faculties/schools of nursing, but also limited understanding of the PHC movement internationally and even of Canada's leadership in promoting PHC through the Ottawa Charter for Health Promotion (1986). Tenn and Niskala (1994) and Rodger and Gallagher (1995) reported encouraging progress with the integration of PHC concepts in basic curricula, but also found problems in developing appropriate practice opportunities to apply the concepts. Some of the difficulties arise from the slowness of change in the health care system from the traditional acute-care orientation to one emphasizing PHC and the health of communities rather than the health of individuals and families. Munro, Herbert, and Murnaghan (1995) have encountered similar problems in developing the new baccalaureate curriculum at the University of Prince Edward Island, which is based on the principles and concepts of PHC. They are endeavouring to create new types of learning opportunities in new environments for students to practice the variety of nursing roles inherent in a PHC framework. As usual with major changes in role expectations within a changing delivery system, "the difficulty is to prepare graduates for current realities, while also providing them with the skills they will require for future practice" (Munro, Herbert, & Murnaghan, 1995, p. 718).

Rodger and Gallagher (1995) reported that one-half of the 25 university nursing faculties/schools that responded to their survey had integrated PHC principles in several courses in the basic program, particularly in community health nursing courses. The PHC principle mentioned most often by respondents was health promotion and disease prevention. This is not surprising since it has been the major principle underlying community health/public health practice for many years. Health promotion and disease prevention was found to be the major thrust of nursing's efforts to promote PHC since enactment of the Canada Health Act in 1984, as reported by the national and provincial/territorial nursing associations responding to Rodger and Callaghan's survey. Nurses have demonstrated for more than a decade that they "are able to play a leadership role in health promotion. They are effective at initiating health education and other activities that assist, promote and support clients as they strive to achieve the highest possible level of health" (CNA, 1995 April, p.2). University faculties/schools of nursing reported that PHC content had been increased in all but one of the basic programs. Some added new courses, such as community development, community assessment, and community health practice with populations; several mentioned the development of new clinical placements congruent with PHC principles. Some of these changes were made in response to the report of The Working Group (1991), who found that basic curricula were not preparing students adequately for the role expectations for community health nurses, as reflected in publications by the Canadian Public Health Association (CPHA). The goal is "to promote and preserve the health of populations and is directed to communities, groups, families and individuals across their lifespan" (CPHA, 1990, p. 3).

If PHC is to become the major focus of nursing practice and nursing education, the 5 principles of PHC—accessibility; health promotion and disease prevention; public participation, intersectoral and interdisciplinary collaboration; and appropriate technology—must be regarded as the foundation of all nursing practice. Hence, the principles need to be integrated in the curriculum from the outset rather than focused in the last year of the program or in selected courses. Programs have been moving away from traditional curriculum patterns and the influence of the medical model; however, the creative use of new and different practice opportunities is needed for students to implement all of the PHC principles in practice. For example, new placements are likely to be needed to permit students to observe and work with individuals and groups designed to facilitate public participation in changing the health care system to better meet their needs. Such experiences might be obtained through nursing associations involved in informing the public and enabling their participation in effecting changes through public service announcements and brochures; in organizing focus groups and discussions on community health problems; in seeking public input in the development of health policy and PHC projects; and in facilitating public involvement in a PHC project established and managed by nurses.

The public participation principle of PHC is defined by CNA (1995 April) as the following:

> Clients should be encouraged to participate in planning and making decisions about their own health care. Nurses increase public participation in health care by:
> - Involving clients in decisions about their own health;
> - Encouraging clients to take action for their own health;
> - Involving clients in identifying their own health needs;
> - Involving clients in planning, using and evaluating their own health care services; and
> - Encouraging and utilizing community development approaches (p.2).

Tenn and Niskala (1994) reported that community participation and empowerment as a strategy to promote participation are concepts rarely included in curricula and that clinical placements are rarely conducive to public participation. New settings need to be sought, such as citizen groups organized for specific purposes; group homes; youth organizations; coalitions for community action, such as HIV/AIDS care, homeless families, hunger centres, and teenage pregnancy; and programs to promote the health of communities. In such placements there should be opportunity to implement most of the principles of PHC.

Tenn and Niskala (1994) reported that "intersectoral collaboration is a PHC principle that seems to be integrated to a reasonable degree in the majority of nursing programs" (p. 3). However, they did not elaborate on the nature of the integration. In contrast, Rodger and Gallagher (1995) found limited evidence of the professional associations' involvement in activities "that promote collaboration outside the traditional health professions and outside the health care system" (p. 47). The only examples they found were at the Registered Nurses Association of British Columbia's participation in bicycle helmet and safe drinking water projects; the Newfoundland nurses' involvement with several community groups in addressing such problems as substance abuse; and Quebec nurses' involvement in multiple-community projects that use intersectoral models. It is important that nursing educators understand the differences between interdisciplinary and intersectoral collaboration. The principle of intersectoral collaboration is described by CNA (1995 April) as:

> Health activities must be undertaken concurrently with measures aimed at improving economic and social development. Professionals from all disciplines should cooperate with each other, with clients, with professionals from other sectors and with governments. Nurses coordinate client care and strive to integrate health services. Nurses also participate with clients in designing healthy public policies and will continue to do so to achieve health for all (p. 2).

With cutbacks in health care funding and services and the recent trends toward privatization of government services, nurses must continue to be concerned about efforts that threaten Canadians' access to essential health services, such as user fees and extra-billing. The principle of accessibility states that:

All Canadians should have reasonable access to essential health services with no financial barriers. Nurses provide more options for accessing health services by:
- Acting as entry point for clients into the health care system;
- Providing nursing care and treatment for health problems;
- Helping clients to identify and use health resources, both formal and informal; and
- Acting as a source of health information for clients (CNA, 1995 April, pp. 1-2).

Throughout the basic curriculum students have many opportunities to implement this principle in a variety of clinical practice settings, with the exception of serving as an entry point. With the innovative projects undertaken by nursing associations, by university faculties/schools of nursing, and by individuals or groups as special projects, there should be opportunities for students to learn about the outcomes of such ventures and for some to observe and/or practice in the settings. Some examples cited by Rodger and Gallagher (1995) are the Cheticamp Primary Health Care Project in Nova Scotia by the Registered Nurses Association of Nova Scotia; the Newfoundland-Denmark PHC Project by the Association of Registered Nurses of Newfoundland; and the Northwest Territories' Rankin Inlet Project by the Northwest Territories Registered Nurses Association. The Increased Direct Access to Services Provided by Registered Nurses Project undertaken by the Alberta Association of Registered Nurses serves as an example from which students could learn approaches to changing the system to utilize nurses appropriately and increase accessibility for clients.

Students are exposed to and have experience with high technology in the course of hospital practice experiences and become aware of issues surrounding the use of high cost, high-tech care. They need to be apprised of the PHC principle pertaining to appropriate technology and their responsibilities in the future for implementing it, as stated in the principle:

> Technology and modes of care should be based on health needs, and appropriately adapted to the community's social, economic and cultural development. There is a need to develop alternatives to high cost, high-tech health care services and make better use of other lower-cost, highly qualified health care providers and services. Nurses provide cost-effective care that is based on client needs, research evidence, and measurable health outcomes. They should be involved in developing, implementing, and evaluating technology and modes of care to ensure their appropriateness and cost-effectiveness (CNA, 1995 April, p.2).

Finding appropriate practice opportunities for nursing students has always presented a challenge to nursing educators. This applies not only to the settings but also to the role models within the settings for students to emulate. This problem has been discussed in the nursing literature for almost three decades by nursing leaders, some of whom have designed and tested strategies to develop the desired role models and the quality of practice students are to emulate. One strategy employed with considerable success is a system of joint appointments between university faculties/schools of nursing and the health care and other community agencies used for students' practice. In a recent survey MacPhail (1996) found that 11 of the 19 faculties/schools from which a response was received, had developed a system of joint appointments (Alberta, British Columbia, Calgary, Dalhousie, McMaster, Ottawa, Toronto, and Victoria). Three other universities (McGill, Queen's, and Saskatchewan) reported offering adjunct appointments in the faculty to selected health-care agency personnel, but no appointments for faculty members in health-care agencies. Most of the 8 respondents who do not have a system of joint appointments indicated interest in them, particularly l'université de Montréal who reported a collaboration model in the process of development (MacPhail, 1996, p. 342).

Preceptorships by well qualified preceptors in health-care agencies is another approach to providing supervision of students and also promoting collaboration between nursing education and nursing practice. Finding preceptors with knowledge and skills in PHC presents another challenge for nursing educators and nursing leaders in health-care agencies. Stewart (1995) points out that "the barriers to widespread implementation of PHC in curricula are identical to those faced in practice (i.e., resources, attitudes, skills, and knowledge) and must be overcome" (p. 780). A collaborative approach to educating both faculty members and agency personnel about PHC offers great potential for nursing to design and test new approaches to applying the principles of PHC in nursing practice and nursing education.

■ Research in Community Health Nursing

The need for increasing nursing research as a basis for practice in community health nursing has been set forth in Chapter 6. Also identified were deterrents to the conduct of research in nursing and possible strategies to overcome them. The challenge to nursing researchers in community health is not only to expand and enhance the quality of nursing research, but also to assess the outcomes of a variety of approaches to implementing the five principles of primary health care (PHC) for the health of Canadians. Of vital importance also is systematic evaluation of the effectiveness of different approaches and teaching strategies as Canadian university faculties/schools of nursing move forward with the integration of the five principles of PHC throughout curricula on both the baccalaureate and graduate levels.

To accomplish these goals will require increased commitment to research by all nurses because of the broad implications of adopting a focus of PHC in nursing. It is envisioned as the means for reaching nursing's potential in achieving health for all Canadians. There is no doubt that the Canadian health care system will change because the costs of the current system far exceed available resources. It is incumbent on nurses to influence the direction and nature of changes to emphasize health care rather than illness care and ensure that this is reflected in funding of both care and research to strengthen the scientific base for care. It is no longer sufficient to profess that PHC is the direction for the future; researchers must provide data that demonstrate the value in terms of health care outcomes and the cost effectiveness of the strategies used. Nurses cannot accomplish this alone; they must implement the PHC principle of public participation to engender the public support in lobbying and developing healthy public policy. Priority should be given to increasing funding for both research and the preparation of researchers through doctoral education. Leaders in nursing education and nursing practice must then ensure that the expectations for the conduct and dissemination of research findings are met and that the research base of practice continues to be strengthened.

Future directions in nursing research need to be directed toward not only increasing the quantity and quality of research, increasing funding and commitment to disseminate findings and facilitate their application in practice, but also to extending the focus of studies from individuals and aggregates to research on communities, groups, and families. There has been a preponderance of individual studies in nursing research rather than replication studies that are needed to increase confidence in research, findings obtained from larger samples. This has implications for the development of public policy as well as for changes in practice. Much of nursing research has involved isolated studies rather than programmatic research, which is needed to build a sufficient body of knowledge about the phenomenon being studied to warrant changes in practice. Programmatic research is more likely to be funded, as reflected in the funding of six research centres in university faculties/schools of nursing by the Medical Research Council of Canada and the National Health Research and Development Program. An example is the research on social support at Dalhousie University School of Nursing, which is designed to: "Assess support experienced by neglected populations; examine the conceptual links among social supports, coping, and self-care; and test the impact of support interventions on health status, health behaviour, and health services use" (Stewart, 1995, p. 89). Client populations included in the studies of social support include mothers of children with cystic fibrosis, diabetes, spina bifida, and with chronic illness; children undergoing stressful health care procedures; persons with ischemic heart disease who are admitted to hospital; persons with cardiac illness and stroke victims and their family caregivers; and persons with hemophilia and HIV/AIDS, their family caregivers, and bereaved family caregivers. In addition, three other assessment studies have been conducted by graduate students; 4 intervention studies by faculty using telephone support groups and peer visitor support in the home have addressed needs identified in the assessment studies; and social support experienced by nurses as caregivers has been studied. This illustrates the possible outcomes of building a program of research that focuses on the study of a phenomenon.

With the increasing movement of health care from the hospital into the community as one means of controlling health care costs, it is incumbent on nursing researchers to assess systematically through research the outcomes for communities, families and population groups, as well as for individuals. The findings are important in developing healthy public policy, that is, policy that will promote the health of families and communities as well as individuals.

Priority should be given to assessing the outcomes of nurses' efforts to make health care more accessible to Canadians by nurses serving as entry points into the healthcare system. These data are needed to help influence changes in the delivery system designed to utilize nurses' talents more effectively as well as increase accessibility to health care. Similarly, the projects undertaken by the provincial/territorial nursing associations should have a sound research component so the outcomes can be used in changing public policy to permit nurses to practise such roles throughout Canada, rather than be limited to isolated areas where physicians choose not to practise. It is important that research methods, including valid and reliable instruments, be shared through publication and research conferences so time and funds are not wasted in designing and testing new assessment tools when reliable instruments are available.

The development of appropriate and scientifically sound research methods to study populations and communities offers a real challenge to nursing researchers in community health. Traditional methods are oriented to individuals primarily and to research conducted in controlled environments, whereas community health nursing practice takes place primarily in naturalistic settings. Traditional quantitative and epidemiological research methods have made major contributions to the study of health problems, and survey methods used commonly in community studies are appropriate for some purposes but provide limited information about the actual practice of community health nurses and its effectiveness in promoting health. Qualitative research methods such as grounded theory, ethnography, and phenomenology are particularly suited to investigating problems in natural settings, which is where community health nurses practise primarily. It is only in recent years that qualitative methods have become more acceptable in nursing research; however, it has been difficult to obtain research funding because the methods are not known and not understood by quantitative researchers who have predominated research review committees on the national level and may even have been discredited by some reviewers (Chalmers & Gregory, 1995). If the research needed to move forward with the implementation of PHC principles is to be done, new research methods may be needed and existing methods particularly suited to the study of communities, populations and families, should be accepted and funded.

Participatory action research is one such method suited to the investigation of problems perceived as critical or priority by the public. This method was first developed in Europe and Canada as part of the healthy cities movement, and there have been more than 400 such initiatives undertaken worldwide since 1986 (Flynn, Rider & Bailey, 1992). The ultimate goal of this strategy is to develop healthy public policy which implies policy decisions with explicit concern for health promotion that have the same priority in planning as economic policy. It focuses on the community, involving residents in every part of the process, including the identification of problems, selection of methods of investigation and of subjects, and even in deciding what to do with the findings. Flynn, Ray and Rider (1994) regard participatory action research as "essential to the community empowerment process. Through dialogue, both researcher and community members grow in their understanding of the phenomena under investigation" (p. 104). They also note that "community groups with the worst health problems often have the least access to community power . . . [and that] community health is promoted by increased citizen participation in the community power structures" (p. 404). This research method seems a logical approach to the investigation of problems arising from the socioeconomic determinants of health, such as poverty, racism, violence, pollution and stigmatization. It has also been found useful in studying the health problems of cultural and ethnic groups, as illustrated by Dickson (1995) in her study of Aboriginal women and by Brunt (1995) in his study of the health problems of Hutterite communities. Brunt (1995) states that "the emerging field of participatory action research holds exciting promise for translating the multifactorial influences on health into positive PHC and health promotion programs" (p. 679). Dickson (1995) expresses concern about the reluctance of traditional researchers and funding agencies to accept this research method. Hopefully, this attitude will change as its value in studying the health problems of communities and population groups are recognized.

In this age of rapidly expanding technology nursing researchers can make an important contribution to the systematic assessment of technologies and thus, help to implement the PHC principle of appropriate technology. They should be involved in developing, implementing, and evaluating technology and modes of care to ensure their appropriateness and their cost-effectiveness.

The sharing of research findings and discussion of research ideas in community health nursing was facilitated by the First International Conference on Community Health Nursing Research, held in Edmonton, Alberta in September 1993 and sponsored by the Edmonton Board of Health. It attracted more than 900 nurses from 40 countries, and included 372 oral presentations of research and 80 poster presentations, as well as plenary sessions presented by eight internationally recognized nursing researchers selected as keynote speakers. Of the 457 abstracts selected for presentation, 45% were Canadian and the remaining 55% were largely from the United States and Europe, although nearly 20% were from Asia, Africa, Australia/New Zealand, and Latin America. Community development and PHC were two topics that received considerable attention from nursing researchers. More than half of the 35 papers on community development were presented by Canadians, but only 6% of the PHC papers were by Canadians; however, Canadians presented 12% of the research in health promotion. In her opening keynote address, Dr. Miriam Hirschfeld, WHO Chief Scientist for Nursing since 1989, "emphasized that health issues are not limited to the domain of nursing, but are shared concerns of the public, relevant professional sectors, and politicians [and] cautioned that narrow research questions, especially those that examine efficiencies, but do not address health outcomes, can be misused on the political agenda." She emphasized the need for good research on obstacles to attaining PHC and the goal of health for all, particularly problems in facilitating public participation (King, Mills, and Stinson, 1995, p. 688). The final keynoter, Dr. Lisbeth Hockey of the United Kingdom, warned researchers against

> conducting irrelevant research; complacency over what has been achieved, when the rhetoric currently surrounding a shift toward community programming may be more fiscally driven than altruistically and/or substantively promoted; territorial possessiveness, which is divisive at a time when sharing is needed, excessive specialization and isolation in an era that warrants generalization and collaboration; and the generation of language that is incomprehensible when clarity is required for communication to occur (King, Mills, and Stinson, 1995, p. 692).

The challenges and opportunities for making a significant contribution to the development of a research base for PHC in Canada are many and varied. Responsibility for assessing the effectiveness of different strategies designed to improve the health of Canadians and implement the principles of PHC, rests with researchers in community health nursing. Community health nurses should pay heed to the admonitions of Hirschfeld and Hockey as they move forward with strengthening the research base for practice toward the goal of Health for All.

■ Summary

The challenges in community health nursing identified in this chapter are exciting and demanding. A revolution is taking place in health care as the traditional system is being questioned on all fronts. The opportunities for the nursing profession in moving into advanced practice roles in community health nursing and in influencing directions that the restructuring process of the health system can take have never been greater. The nursing profession has accomplished a great deal in its three-and-a-half centuries in Canada. There is no doubt that even greater accomplishments are yet to be seen. In all areas of nursing practice, education, administration, and research, current issues in community health nursing are front and centre in discussions of health reform. It is essential for every nurse to develop an awareness of matters of professional significance in community health nursing, for these affect everyday practice. The nursing profession has a great deal to offer to discussions of the shift to the community, for its members have decades of experience in serving as key professionals in implementing strategies designed to improve health in the community.

REFERENCES

Brunt, J.H. (1995). Epidemiology in community health nursing: Principles and applications for primary health care. In M.J. Stewart (Ed.), *Community nursing: Promoting Canadians' health* (pp. 662-682). Toronto: W.B. Saunders.

Canadian Nurses Association. (1988). *Health for all Canadians—A call for health care reform.* Ottawa, Ontario: The Association.

Canadian Nurses Association. (1995). *Policy statement: The role of the nurse in primary health care.* Ottawa: The Association.

Canadian Nurses Association. (1980). *Putting health into health care.* Ottawa, Ontario: The Association.

Canadian Public Health Association. (1990). *Community health/public health nursing in Canada: Preparation and practice.* Ottawa: The Association.

Chalmers, K.I., & Gregory, D.M. (1995). Community health nursing research: Theoretical and practical challenges. In M.J. Stewart (Ed.), *Community nursing: Promoting Canadians' health* (pp. 600-617). Toronto: W.B. Saunders.

Dickson, G. (1995). Participatory action research: Theory and practice. In M.J. Stewart (Ed.), *Community nursing: Promoting Canadians' health* (pp. 640-661). Toronto: W.B. Saunders.

Edwards, N.C., & Craig, H. (1987). *Does nursing education reflect the goals of primary health care?* Hamilton, Ontario: McMaster University.

Flynn, B.C., Ray, D.W., & Rider, M.S. (1994). Empowering communities: Action research through healthy cities. *Health Education Quarterly, 21*(3), 395-405.

Flynn, B.C., Rider, M.S., & Bailey, W.W. (1992). Developing community leadership in healthy cities: The Indiana model. *Nursing Outlook, 40*(3), 121-126.

King, M.E., Mills, K.M., & Stinson, S.M. (1995). The first international conference on community health nursing research. In M.J. Stewart (Ed.), *Community nursing: Promoting Canadians' health* (pp. 683-707). Toronto: W.B. Saunders.

MacPhail, J. (1996). Collaboration between nursing education and nursing practice for quality nursing care, education, and research. In J. Ross Kerr & J. MacPhail, *Canadian nursing: Issues and perspectives* (3rd ed) (pp. 334-349). St. Louis: Mosby–Year Book, Inc.

Mahler, H. (1985). Nurses lead the way. *WHO Features* (No. 97). Geneve, Switzerland: World Health Organization.

Munro, M.F., Herbert, R., & Murnaghan, D.A. (1995). Primary health care as a framework for excellence in education. In M.J. Stewart (Ed.), *Community nursing: Promoting Canadians' health* (pp. 710-724). Toronto: W.B. Saunders.

Rodger, J.L., & Gallagher, S.M. (1995). The move toward primary health care in Canada: Community health nursing from 1985 to 1995. In M.J. Stewart (Ed.), *Community nursing: Promoting Canadians' health* (pp. 37-58). Toronto: W.B. Saunders.

Stewart, M.J. (1995). Community health nursing in the future. In M.J. Stewart (Ed.), *Community nursing: Promoting Canadians' health* (pp. 762-788). Toronto: W.B. Saunders.

Stewart, M.J. (1995). Social support, coping, and self-care: Public participation concepts. In M.J. Stewart (Ed.), *Community nursing: Promoting Canadians' health* (pp. 89-124). Toronto: W.B. Saunders.

Stewart, M.J. (1995). The move toward Primary Health Care in Canada: Community health nursing from 1985 to 1995. *Community health nursing: Promoting Canadians' health* (pp. 37-58). Toronto: W.B. Saunders.

Tenn, L., & Niskala, H. (1994). *Primary health care in the curricula of Canadian university schools of nursing.* (Final report to the Canadian Nurses' Foundation). Vancouver: University of British Columbia School of Nursing.

Working Group. (1991). *Report of the Working Group on the educational requirements of community health nurses.* Cat. No. H39-235/1991E. Ottawa: Minister of Supply and Services.

World Health Organization. (1978). *Primary health care: Report on the International Conference on Primary Health Care, Alma-Ata, USSR.* Geneva, Switzerland: WHO.

INDEX

A

Aberdeen, Lady Ishbell, visiting nursing and, 12-13
Abortion as ethical dilemma, 75
Accessibility of services
   in basic undergraduate curriculum, 106-107
   Boyle-McCauley Health Centre and, 49
   financial barriers to, removing, 50-51
   public health care and, 46
Advance directives as ethical dilemmas, 73-75
AFNR; *see* Alberta Foundation for Nursing Research
Aggregates in community health nursing, 82
Alberta
   Public Health Amendment Act in, 100
   task force on primary health care in, 37-38
Alberta Foundation for Nursing Research (AFNR) as funding source for nursing research, 88
Alma-Ata conference, primary health care and, 46
Autonomy, ethics and, 61

B

Battery, consent to nursing care and, 67
Beneficence, ethics and, 61
BMHC; *see* Boyle-McCauley Health Centre
Boyle-McCauley Health Centre (BMHC), 49
British Columbia Children's Hospital, Research Division of, as funding source for nursing research, 88

C

Canada
  health care system of, change in, 41-42
  legal system of, overview of, 62-63
Canada Health Act of 1984, 20
Canadian Nurses Association (CNA)
  challenge of primary health care system and, 34-35
  code of ethics adopted by, 65
  in promoting research and research-based practice, 91
  public health care and, 46
Canadian Nurses' Foundation (CNF) as funding source for nursing research, 87-88
Canadian Nurses Protective Society (CNPS), 70-71
Canadian Red Cross Society, 11-12
Caregivers of cognitively impaired elderly, research on, 83-84
Case law, 62
Centretown Community Health Centre, 48
Childbearing, ethical issues in, 75
Civil law, 62
Class, socioeconomic, in development of public health services, 1-2
Clients' rights, 63-67
Clinical nurse researcher on staff in promoting research and research-based practice, 91-92
CNA; *see* Canadian Nurses Association
CNF; *see* Canadian Nurses' Foundation
CNPS; *see* Canadian Nurses Protective Society
Collaboration; *see also* Cooperation, intersectoral
  development of, as public health care issue, 53-54
  with physicians, 68-69
Communities, health of, primary health care and, 29-44
Community health nursing
  challenges in, 97-112
  future of, 27
  research in, 82-85, 108-112
    epidemiological, 110
    participatory action, 110-111
    programmatic, 109
    qualitative methods of, 110
    quantitative, 110
    sharing findings of, 111-112
Community health nursing practice, education for, 102-108
Complementary model of nursing practice in primary health care, 35-36
Computerization, nursing documentation and, 69-70

Confidentiality
    clients' right to respect and, 64
    ethics and, 61
    as legal issue, 68
Consent to nursing care, 67-68
Constitutional responsibility for health, 16-17
Cooperation, intersectoral
    in basic undergraduate curriculum, 106
    Boyle-McCauley Health Centre and, 49
    in public health care, nursing education and, 54-55
    public health care and, 47
    public health nursing and, 48
    Victorian Order of Nurses and, 49

D

Death, right to make choices in relation to, 66-67
Deontological approaches to ethical issues, 61
Directives, advance, as ethical dilemmas, 73-75
"Do not resuscitate" orders as ethical dilemmas, 71-73
Documentation, nursing, 69-70

E

Education
    for community health nursing practice, 102-108
        curriculum for, basic undergraduate, primary health care concepts in, 104-108
    nursing
        ethics teaching in, 78-79
        implications of public health care for, 54-57
        in promoting research and research-based practice, 90-91
Enacted law, 62
Environments, healthy, achieving, 31-32
Ethical dilemmas
    in health care, 71-77
    strategies for addressing, 77-79
Ethical issues
    childbearing, 75
    deontological approaches to, 61
    ecological survival and, 59
    health-care resource allocation as, 75-77
    increased complexity of, factors contributing to, 60
    in nursing practice, 59-79
    rationing of health care as, 75-77

Ethical issues—cont'd
  teleological approaches to, 61
Ethical principles, basic, 60-62
Ethical theories, basic, 60-62
Ethics
  autonomy and, 61
  beneficence and, 61
  code of, 64-66
  confidentiality and, 61
  definition of, 60
  justice and, 61
  nonmaleficence and, 61
  paternalism and, 61
  personhood and, 61
  veracity and, 61
Ethics committees, 78
Euthanasia, 66-67

F

Facility fees, 20
Family health, primary health care and, 46-57
Fiscal Arrangements and Established Programs Financing Act of 1977, 19-20
Funding sources for nursing research, 87-89

G

Geographic location, health and, 40
Grey Nuns of Montreal, 6-8

H

Hébert, Mme Marie, 2
Hand-washing instruction for children, research on, 82-83
Hôtel Dieu of Quebec, founding of, 3-4
Health
  for all, Canadian approach to achieving, 30-32
  of communities, primary health care and, 29-44
  concept of, broadening of, as public health care issue, 52-53
  constitutional responsibility for, 16-17
  definition of, nursing education and, 54
  as focus of health services, 32
  socioeconomic determinants of, 39-41
Health care
  accessibility of, 21
  in Canada, shape and structure of, 16-27

Health care—cont'd
  comprehensiveness of, 21
  human rights in, 63-64
  nurses as access to, 49-50
  portability of, 21
  primary, 33-34
    World Health Organization vision of, 101
  principles of, 21
  public administration of, 21
  rationing of, as ethical dilemma, 75-77
  reform of, 22
  universality of, 21
Health care reform movement, 98-99
Health care services, essential determining, as public health care issue, 51
Health for All by the Year 2000, 29-30
Health system, restructuring of, 98-99
Health-care resources, allocation of, as ethical dilemma, 75-77
History, 1-15
Hospital Insurance and Diagnostic Services Act of 1957, 18
Hospitalières de la Micéricorde de Jésus, 3-8
    Grey Nuns of Montreal and, 6-8
    Jeanne Mance and, 4-5

I

ICN; *see* International Council of Nurses
Informed, clients' right to be, 63
Insurance, liability, for nurses, Canadian Nurses Protective Society and, 70-71
International Council of Nurses (ICN), primary health care and, 29-30
Intersectoral cooperation, public health care and, 47

J

Judicial system, 62
Justice, ethics and, 61

L

La Société de Notre Dame de Jésus, 4-5
Law
  case versus enacted, 62
  civil versus public, 62
  nurses' actions under, 67-71
Lay participation in public health care, 46-47
    nursing education and, 54-55
Leadership, nursing, opportunities for, in primary health care, 42-43

Legal issues in nursing practice, 59-79
Legal responsibilities of nurses, 63
Legal system, Canadian, overview of, 62-63
Liability insurance for nurses, Canadian Nurses Protective Society and, 70-71
Living wills, 74

M

Mack School, 11
Mance, Jeanne, 4-5
Manitoba, primary health care initiatives in, 36
McAdam Project in New Brunswick, nurses' role in, 49-50
McGill model of nursing, 55-57
Medical Care Insurance Act of 1966, 19
Medical Research Council (MRC) as funding source for nursing research, 87
Medicare
    evolution of, 17-21
        Canada Health Act of 1984 in, 20
        facility fees and, 20
        Fiscal Arrangements and Established Programs Financing Act of 1977 in, 19-20
        Hospital Insurance and Diagnostic Services Act of 1957 in, 18
        Medical Care Insurance Act of 1966 in, 19
        National Health Grants Act of 1948 in, 18
    federal funding for, impending loss of, 20-21
    philosophical basis of, 21-22
    threats to, 23-26
        maldistribution of physicians as, 25
        misuse of system as, 24
        resource limitations as, 23-24
        underutilization of nurses as, 25-26
MRC; *see* Medical Research Council

N

National Council of Women, 1-2
National Health Grants Act of 1948, 18
Negligence, 70
New France, nursing in, 2-3
Newfoundland
    primary health care initiatives in, 36
    primary health care project in, 37
Nightingale, Florence, 10
Nonmaleficence, ethics and, 61
Nurse(s)
    as access to health care, 49-50

Nurse(s)—cont'd
　appropriate use of
　　basic undergraduate curriculum and, 107-108
　　as public health care issue, 51-52
　education of
　　ethics teaching in, 78-79
　　implications of public health care for, 54-57
　　in promoting research and research-based practice, 90-91
　legal responsibilities of, 63
　prepared to conduct research, limited number of, 85
　in primary health care, 33-34
　public health, 47-48
　role of, in health care, physicians and, 100-102
　underutilization of, as threat to Medicare, 25-26
Nursing
　documentation in, 69-70
　ethical and legal questions in, 59-79
　leadership in, opportunities for, in primary health care, 42-43
　McGill model of, 55-57
　in New France, 2-3
　response of, to challenge of primary health care system, 34-39
　visiting, 12-15
Nursing care, consent to, 67-68
Nursing practice
　professional, changing focus of, 99-102
　research-based, 81-82
　　deterrents to, 85-90
　　　access to clients as, 87
　　　difficulty in asking research question as, 85-86
　　　funding limitations as, 87-89
　　　limited number of nurses prepared to conduct research as, 85
　　　time constraints as, 86-87
　　　utilization of research findings in practice settings as, 89-90
　　future of, 95
　　strategies to promote, 90-95

O

Ontario, primary health care initiatives in, 36-37
Ontario Ministry of Health as funding source for nursing research, 88
Ottawa, primary health care initiatives in, 36

P

Paternalism, ethics and, 61

Personhood, ethics and, 61
Personnel, appropriate use of, as public health care issue, 51-52
PHC; *see* Primary health care
Physician(s)
    collaboration with, 68-69
    maldistribution of, as threat to Medicare, 25
    nurses' role in health care and, 100-102
Populations, underserved, outreach to, centres with, 48-49
Poverty, health and, 39-40
Prepaid hospital care, legislation on, 18
Prepaid medical care, legislation on, 19
Preventive/promotive care
    Boyle-McCauley Health Centre and, 49
    nurses role in, evolution of, 97-99
    public health care and, 46
    public health nursing and, 47-48
    Victorian Order of Nurses and, 49
Primary health care (PHC)
    in Canada, current examples of, 47-50
    challenge of, nursing's response to, 34-39
    concepts of, in basic undergraduate curriculum, 104-108
    family health and, 46-57
    future of, 43-44
    health of communities and, 29-44
    nurse in, 33-34
    nursing leadership opportunities in, 42-43
Private law, 62
Public health
    emerging concept of, 8-10
Public Health Amendment Act, 100
Public health care
    concepts of, in basic undergraduate curriculum, 104-108
    issues in, 50-54
        appropriate use of personnel as, 51-52
        broadening concept of health as, 52-53
        collaboration development as, 53-54
        determining essential services as, 51
        removing financial barriers to accessible health care as, 50-51
    McGill model of nursing and, 55-57
    nurses as access to health care in, 49-50
    nursing education and, 54-57
    principles of, 46
Public health nursing in modern context, 10-15

Public health nursing services, 47-48
Public law, 62

R

Replacement model of nursing practice in primary health care, 35
Research
   community health nursing, 82-85
   in community health nursing, 108-112
      epidemiological, 110
      participatory action, 110-111
      programmatic, 109
      qualitative methods of, 110
      quantitative, 110
      sharing findings of, 111-112
   consultation on, in promoting research and research-based practice, 92-93
   nurses prepared to conduct, limited number of, 85
   nursing, as basis for community health nursing practice, 81-95
   nursing practice based on, 81-82; *see* Nursing practice, research-based
      deterrents to, 85-90
   strategies to promote, 90-95
   summaries of, in promoting research-based practice, 93
Research committee in health care agency in promoting research and research-based practice, 93
Research Division of British Columbia Children's Hospital as funding source for nursing research, 88
Research interest groups in promoting research and research-based practice, 94
Research question, difficulty in asking, 85-86
Research roundtable discussions, unit-based, in promoting research and research-based practice, 93
Resources, health-care, allocation of, as ethical dilemma, 75-77
Respect, clients' right to, 63-64
Right(s)
   clients,' 63-67
   human, in health care, 63-64
   to make choices in relation to death, 66-67
Rollet, Marie, 2

S

Saskatchewan, early health care in, 17-18
Self-care in health promotion, 31
Self-determination, clients' right to, 64
Socioeconomic determinants of health, 39-41
Socioeconomic status in development of public health services, 1-2

Stigmatized populations, health and, 40-41

T

Technology, appropriate
  in basic undergraduate curriculum, 107
  public health care and, 47
Teleological approaches to ethical issues, 61
Telephone orders, validation of, 68-69

V

Veracity, ethics and, 61
Victorian Order of Nurses (VON), 1
  as funding source for nursing research, 88
  public health care and, 49
  public health nursing and, 11-12
  visiting nursing and, 13
Visiting nursing, 12-15
VON; *see* Victorian Order of Nurses

W

Wills, living, 74
Women in development of public health services, 1-2